My Quest for Health Equity

HEALTH EQUITY IN AMERICA

Daniel E. Dawes, Series Editor

My Quest
for Health Equity

Notes on Learning While Leading

DAVID SATCHER, MD, PhD

Johns Hopkins University Press
Baltimore

Johns Hopkins University Press
2715 North Charles Street
Baltimore, Maryland 21218-4363
www.press.jhu.edu

Library of Congress Cataloging-in-Publication Data

Names: Satcher, David, 1941– author.
Title: My quest for health equity : notes on learning while leading / David
    Satcher, MD, PhD.
Description: Baltimore : Johns Hopkins University Press, 2020. | Series: Health
    equity in America | Includes bibliographical references and index.
Identifiers: LCCN 2019041634 | ISBN 9781421438313 (hardcover ; alk. paper) |
    ISBN 9781421438320 (ebook)
Subjects: MESH: Satcher, David, 1941– | Health equity | Leadership | Public
    health | United States | Personal narrative
Classification: LCC RA418 | NLM W 76 AA1 | DDC 362.1—dc23
LC record available at https://lccn.loc.gov/2019041634

A catalog record for this book is available from the British Library.

*Special discounts are available for bulk purchases of this book. For more information,
please contact Special Sales at specialsales@press.jhu.edu.*

Johns Hopkins University Press uses environmentally friendly book materials,
including recycled text paper that is composed of at least 30 percent post-
consumer waste, whenever possible.

I am pleased to dedicate this book to my late wife Nola Richardson Satcher, who died on June 23, 2019, after living with Alzheimer's disease for more than twenty years. Nola was a beautiful lady with a beautiful spirit, and I was fortunate to be married to her for forty years. We married two years after my first wife, Callie, the mother of my four children, died of breast cancer in 1978. Nola adopted our children, who were then between the ages of one and nine.

Nola was a poet and took seriously the rhythm of life, which most of us ignore or miss completely. During our forty years together, she supported me in all of my endeavors. She served as first lady of Meharry Medical College for almost twelve years; she served as first lady of the CDC; in the Office of the Surgeon General; and as the first lady of Morehouse School of Medicine. During most of these years and in the positions in which she served, she was struggling with Alzheimer's, a disease that had also led to her mother's death in 2003.

I owe Nola more than I could ever say, and I will always love her dearly.

Contents

Acknowledgments

I hope that I have written this book in a way that is in and of itself an acknowledgment of the tremendous contribution my parents and siblings made to my survival and development. Dr. Jackson, who saved my life when I was two years old, died before I had a chance to meet him. He visited our small farm on his off day as I struggled with whooping cough and pneumonia. By not being able to admit me to the local hospital, Dr. Jackson was a victim of the same racist system that placed me at such great risk. I will always be grateful to him and for his dedication to medicine. I hope I have lived and continue to live my life in a way that brings honor to Dr. Jackson, my family, and all of those who have contributed to my almost eighty years of life.

This book is also a tribute to the great support I have received during the process of writing and advancing this topic. I especially want to express my appreciation to my assistant, Mrs. Yvonne Kirkland, who has been committed to helping to make my work a reality and has always been concerned about the quality and relevance of my work.

Dr. Joyce H. Nottingham and I met when I was a senior at Morehouse College and she was at Spelman College. I was a teaching assistant in the Comparative Anatomy Laboratory, and it was there that I came to appreciate her thirst for learning. I was fortunate when I returned to Atlanta and to Morehouse School of Medicine to find that Dr. Nottingham was still very much involved here. She served as my special assistant when I was president of the school of medicine and later as associate director of the Satcher Health Leadership Institute. I sought and received her assistance in writing this book, and she has done so much to assure its integrity and quality. Special thanks to her for her expertise, diligence, and commitment.

There are many people whom I could thank, but generally I want to express my appreciation to those who value my work and who are willing to strive to make it what it has the potential to be— my greatest hope for the future.

My Quest for Health Equity

Introduction

T HIS IS A BOOK about leadership. I have had the opportunity not only to lead but also to sit at the feet of great
leaders and to take on the challenge and burden of leadership in
academia, community, and government. This book is about a leadership journey that has taken place over a fifty-year period, about
lessons learned while on that journey. Finally, over the last ten
years, I have been involved in developing the Satcher Health Leadership Institute at Morehouse School of Medicine (SHLI/MSM) to
provide support for others who are working to develop their leadership skills.

This book is not intended to be specifically about me. However,
unavoidably, it builds on my life experiences, from the other side of
the track and serving in several critical leadership roles. My inten-
tion is to share what I have learned and am learning in the quest to
achieve public health equity, as well as what we at SHLI/MSM have

learned about developing leaders in this arena. This is for me both a personal goal and a leadership goal. But it is not just about my experience and learning; it is also about those key people who most influenced me and my leadership style, and our shared goal of global health equity.

This is a three-dimensional perspective on leadership. The first dimension is that of a follower who experienced great role models for leadership, beginning with parents who had less than an elementary school education but were great leaders nevertheless; a college president who was dynamic and committed; and a global leader, who led a movement that I joined and who was assassinated at a young age. So the first dimension of my perspective on leadership is dynamic, challenging, and motivational. I was motivated to serve wherever I could contribute to the mission of health equity. Like the book, the first dimension is more the "why" of leadership than the "how."

The second dimension of my leadership perspective came with my assumption of leadership roles in the Atlanta University Center civil rights student movement in the early 1960s. This was the beginning of a lifetime of mission-oriented leadership for me. As I served in various leadership roles, I learned as much about leadership from persons who worked with me and under me as I did from those above me. This was especially true of lessons learned from members of my leadership teams. Leadership is indeed not position dependent, and I have seen great leadership take place at many different levels.

The third dimension derives from my work over the last ten years helping others to develop their leadership skills, while serving as the founding director and senior advisor of the Satcher Health Leadership Institute at Morehouse School of Medicine, and later just as an advisor. Certainly, for these last ten years of my career-life, I've had more time and motivation to focus on the meaning and significance of leadership in my own life and in the lives of others, whether they were health professionals interested in learning how to develop and influence policy; potential community health leaders wanting to enhance their skills and improve community health; or determined (usually single) parents wanting to give their very young children (0 to 5 years) the best start in life. The unofficial motto of SHLI/MSM is that in order to eliminate disparities in health and achieve health equity, we need leaders who care enough, know enough, have the courage to do enough, and who will persevere until the job is done. From my near-death experience as a child in segregated Alabama, to the opportunities I have had to serve in key leadership roles, my personal history and background are certainly relevant to the topic of health equity dealt with in this book.

The common thread running through all three dimensions of my leadership perspective is mission: the "why" of leadership. For my parents, there was a determination that their children would not only survive but would have opportunities that they did not have and would stand for something based on their faith in God. Thus, service to God and others seemed to be my parents' major motivation, and they wanted their children to be much better prepared for this mission than they were. Even though they were suppressed by racial discrimination, which they felt they had to tolerate, they imagined and envisioned a different world for their children, and they wanted us to be prepared for it. My parents were leaders not only in the home but also in the church and community. Much of my perspective on leadership is based on my observation and interaction with them. They truly cared about their children, their community, their church, and their country.

My parents taught me the importance of shared responsibilities. Each one of my siblings and I had jobs, which changed as we grew and developed. My first job was taking water to my siblings in the field. Next, I had the added responsibility of feeding the chickens and other yard animals. This progression continued until I, my-self, was working in the fields chopping cotton, corn, and other crops. Then I had the job of milking the cow and plowing the mule. Our jobs grew in complexity as we grew and aged, but at each stage of work, we were taught how to do the job, and then our work was inspected. In short, our parents believed, "You cannot expect that which you don't inspect." Their inspection was a lesson in learning and leadership.

My parents also were very religious and engaged us in church every Sunday, including Sunday school, where my dad was super-intendent for twenty-five years. Their religion was not just about the Bible and worship, but it included a relationship with their fel-low men and women. I remember our sharing whatever we had (usu-ally meager) with our neighbors when they were in need. If a neigh-bor's cow was not giving milk, and ours was, we shared our milk with them. I remember many times carrying pails of milk to a neigh-bor's home.

I was born in Anniston, Alabama, in 1941. Anniston is located approximately eighty-nine miles from Atlanta, Georgia. The 1940 Census estimated the population to be 25,523 people,[1] and accord-ing to *The Encyclopedia of Alabama*,[2] at that time, one-third of the population was African American. Strict racial segregation became the norm during the 1890s and lasted until the mid-1960s.

At the age of two, I suffered from whooping cough, which led to pneumonia. I was seriously ill, and I can remember struggling to breathe. Dr. Jackson, the one black doctor in the area agreed, after my father's pleading, to come see me on his off day. He spent the entire day with me, and as he prepared to leave, he told my parents that he did not expect me to survive the week. Nevertheless, he told them what they should do to keep me comfortable and give me the best chance of survival. Even though he considered me to be near death, Dr. Jackson could not admit me to the hospital because the only hospital in the area did not admit black patients or allow black physicians to admit. Black kids with illnesses like mine usually died at home, without the benefit of hospital care.

It is clear that I was introduced to disparities in health care early on while living on that forty-four-acre rocky farm outside of Anniston. I survived in great part because my parents believed in God, and while they trusted the physician, their faith led them to believe they could help me through this illness. As was customary, people from the small farm community gathered around, and I could hear them singing and praying while they sat on the front porch. I remember struggling to breathe in the rhythmic whooping cough manner. Even though my mother followed Dr. Jackson's instructions carefully, she occasionally had to breathe for me, while sitting with me throughout the night.

Well, I survived, and my mother recounted that story to me almost every day for the next few years. By the time I was five years old, more than anything, I wanted to meet Dr. Jackson—the man who had helped to save my life. My parents finally agreed to take me to town to meet him for my sixth birthday. Regrettably, Dr. Jackson suffered a stroke and died, at the age of fifty-four, before I had a chance to meet him.

A lasting curiosity about my illness and Dr. Jackson led me to want to be a doctor, "just like Dr. Jackson." Clearly, I didn't understand what that meant; no one in my family had even finished high school. But I was as certain as I had been about anything in my short life that I would become a doctor. I declared it at age six, and the rest is history. By the time I was six years old, I was shaping my mission to contribute to quality health care for all, and ultimately to health equity. That mission has driven me throughout my life and career, and has driven me to write this book.

Leadership for me has never been about a position, even though I have occupied many. Rather, it is about the opportunity and responsibility to move the needle toward health equity. Our work at SHLI/MSM, helping to develop leaders, is directly tied to our commitment to the elimination of disparities in health and the achievement of health equity.

In many ways, my family and I were victims of poverty and racism, but as a college student (1959–1963) during the civil rights and student sit-in movements,[3,4] I had the opportunity to confront racism nonviolently. That experience is certainly a part of who I am. In addition, my history is one of confrontation, of experiencing disparities in health, and of embracing the goal of health equity. Having been born black and poor in the deep South, I was a victim of an unjust health care system; however, I was not unlike hundreds of thousands of other American citizens. The social conditions that were dominant during that time were those that characterized much of America's history of race relations and social inequity.

Discrimination in education, employment, and income, coupled with violence and threats of violence, led to persistent poverty, social exclusion, ignorance, and little or no access to health care. This described the woeful plight of African Americans in much of America, but especially those living under the laws of Jim Crow in the South, especially in Alabama, my home state.

These conditions could only be addressed by a momentous and courageous social commitment of conscience, spirit, blood, sweat, and tears. The civil rights movement has been called the most significant human rights movement in history, and I was there, participating, in the late 1950s and early 1960s as a student leader at Morehouse College in Atlanta. In the process of helping to lead change, I was changed in a way that would propel me into the future.

As a student at Morehouse, I moved from being a victim of racism to having an opportunity to confront racism and segregation. Early in my tenure as a student, a meeting was called by Atlanta University Center student leaders to announce a planned student sit-in movement at restaurants, similar to ones in North Carolina and Mississippi. It would be a nonviolent protest; we would resist the temptation to fight back and would go to jail if necessary. It was clear that we would probably be arrested, with no assurance of how or when we would be released, even though there were lawyers volunteering to work with us. By that time, I had heard Dr. Martin Luther King Jr. speak about nonviolent resistance, so I understood the concept. Given what I had experienced and what my parents had gone through in Alabama, I needed this opportunity to fight back—to confront racism. Despite my anxiety about the impact this could have on my attending medical school, I decided to join the student sit-in movement in 1960. Confronting racism was high on my list of priorities.

One of my favorite Martin Luther King Jr. quotes is "Until a person finds something for which he is willing to die, then he is not fit to live." I was not quite ready to die, but I was ready to risk my cherished career in order to help change the segregation laws and ways of the South.

Student leaders were impressive also. I especially remember three of these upperclassmen. Lonnie King was a junior from Atlanta, and he was especially committed to changing Atlanta, where only black restaurants would serve blacks, and where the largest downtown department store would hire blacks only for menial jobs.

Then there was Marian Wright, now Marian Wright Edelman, a junior at Spelman College, our sister institution. Dynamic and courageous, she spoke with authority. Marian would go on to law school at Yale and become the first black member of the Mississippi Bar. She went on to found the Children's Defense Fund,[5] spending a lifetime fighting for the rights of children in Washington, DC. But first we had to fight the battle of Atlanta.

Another impressive student leader was Otis Moss Jr., who had just graduated from Morehouse College, but was a student in the

Morehouse School of Religion. Otis was dynamic, and would go on to pastor two great churches, including Olivet Institutional Baptist Church in Cleveland, where I would attend medical school. He would also chair the board of trustees at Morehouse College. He was twice selected as one of "America's 15 Greatest Black Preachers" by *Ebony* magazine.[6]

What these three student leaders had in common was a caring and commitment to the cause of justice. I was motivated to follow them and was soon arrested when we sought service at a restaurant in downtown Atlanta, and later at other segregated establishments.

We were well prepared physically and mentally for what we had to face. We knew how to fall and to protect our faces and heads; we pushed each other downstairs in order to prepare to fall properly; and when we were out on the picket line, we anticipated and dealt with the attacks that came to us without striking back. For us, non-violence was a real commitment.

On Sundays, a group of fellow students and I would walk four to five miles to downtown Atlanta, to Ebenezer Baptist Church, where Dr. King was co-pastor with his father. Whenever we knew Dr. King was in town and preaching, we would set out, after attending the required chapel service at Morehouse College, to make it in time to hear Dr. King preach. Dr. King had the most unusual ability to *educate*, *motivate*, and *mobilize* people to action, and he certainly motivated me and others to join the student movement.

In many ways, both Dr. King and I were motivated by a common leader. Dr. Benjamin Elijah Mays, the president of Morehouse College from 1940 to 1967, was committed to academic excellence for every student who entered the school. He spoke in chapel every Tuesday morning, and we sat on the edge of our seats as he challenged us to "aim for the stars, and not the ceilings of your lives." He did not encourage us to go to jail, but his message was clear: we shouldn't accept less than the best from ourselves or society. Later, speaking at my inauguration as the new president of Meharry Medical College in 1982, Dr. Mays was in a wheelchair, but he repeated that challenge to me and Meharry, and we listened to him. Martin Luther King Jr. heard that message when he was a Morehouse student in the late 1940s, and I heard it as a student in the early 1960s.

My favorite Benjamin Elijah Mays quote, which I have carried with me throughout my life and work, is as follows:

> It must be borne in mind that the tragedy of life doesn't lie in not reaching your goal. The tragedy lies in having no goal to reach. It isn't a calamity to die with dreams unfulfilled, but it is a calamity not to dream. It is not a disaster to be unable to capture your ideal, but it is a disaster to have no ideal to capture. It is not a disgrace not to reach the stars, but it is a disgrace to have no stars to reach for. Not failure, but low aim is sin.[7]

Dr. Mays motivated me to work to achieve excellence and not be happy with less than my best. So, despite my involvement in the student movement, I took my studies seriously, even taking my books to jail with me. I excelled in the classroom, graduating magna cum laude. On one occasion, I emerged from jail just in time to take a biochemistry exam the next day; it was somewhat unnerving. But when we got our grades, I learned I had made the second highest score on the exam. While that felt good to me, my classmate who had made the highest score didn't think very much of someone who would go to jail and come back and not do his best on the exam. There is more than one perspective to every story, and in this case, I got the benefit of both perspectives.

My own leadership would also begin at Morehouse College, where I was elected and served as Student Government Association president during my senior year. I would also rise to leadership of the student movement, when we spent a week in jail on a hunger strike. This strike, which was widely publicized, led business leaders in the community to come together and say that if Atlanta was going to become a global city, it couldn't afford this kind of publicity. We agreed. Thus, the process of desegregation began and grew.

I have been a victim of racism and segregation, and as a student, I have had the opportunity to confront racism. And as a student, I also became a leader, and would leave for medical school at Case Western Reserve in Ohio, knowing that I had the responsibility to see myself not just as a victim but as one who confronted racism, and as a leader in medicine. It should be noted that when I left college to go to medical school, most hospitals in the South would not allow black physicians to admit patients. In fact, it was in 1964 in Greensboro, North Carolina, that the case was brought that forced hospitals who wanted to receive Medicaid and Medicare funding to end discrimination. In time, it virtually ended that kind of discrimination throughout the country.

The student sit-in movement motivated me to be not just a doctor but a leader in medicine, as well. When I left college and headed to medical school, I had both a passion for and a commitment to leadership.

Over the course of my life, I have had many opportunities to lead. I have been a leader in academia, as president of two medical colleges; within churches; as director of a major governmental public health agency; and as surgeon general and assistant secretary for health of the United States of America. In spite of this, I do not consider myself an expert in leadership. Instead, I regard myself as a serious student of leadership, which I see as a continuous learning process. I agree with President John F. Kennedy's November 22, 1963, undelivered statement for the Dallas Trade Mart: "Leadership and learning are indispensable to each other."[8]

Over the years, I would have many opportunities to lead, and fourteen years ago, the Morehouse School of Medicine Board of Trustees voted to establish the Satcher Health Leadership Institute. I felt that I had a lot to share with students of leadership, as I continued to learn myself. But it was the mission of striving for and achieving health equity that motivated me, from my near-death experience in Alabama until this day, as I seek to help others to become the best leaders that they can be.

My major focus today, through SHLI/MSM, is on developing future leaders who will work to close the gaps in life expectancy, infant mortality, and cancer mortality rates between minorities, especially African Americans, and the majority population. To do this, new leaders must be prepared to effect critical public policy decisions, including improvements in access to quality health care, and health promotion and disease prevention, with the goal of eliminating disparities in health and achieving health equity.

Work to establish a leadership development institute was begun in June 2006, when the Satcher Health Leadership Institute formally opened at the Morehouse School of Medicine in Atlanta. The mission of the institute is to develop a diverse group of exceptional leaders, advance and support comprehensive health-systems strategies, and actively promote policies and practices that will ultimately eliminate disparities in health. Like me, the SHLI is driven by the "why" of leadership rather than the "how." We are on a mission.

While other health leadership programs have a minor focus on diversity and inclusion in leadership, SHLI/MSM is the only health leadership organization to make the elimination of health disparities its primary focus and to encourage underrepresented minorities to take advantage of opportunities to provide service and leadership in improving health equity and eliminating health disparities. The fact that SHLI/MSM provides leadership development programs for health professionals and community health leaders, and programs in quality parenting, makes it unique in its relevance and to the goal of health equity.

After having served nine years in government as director of the Centers for Disease Control and Prevention (CDC) and as the sixteenth United States surgeon general and assistant secretary for health, I joined the MSM, in September 2002, to develop the National Center for Primary Care. Two years later, during an institutional crisis, the MSM Board of Trustees and faculty asked me to assume the role of interim president. I agreed to do so.

While serving as interim president (December 2004–July 2006), I initiated an effort to enhance the institution's quality of leadership and leadership preparedness. In part, my motivation was selfish because I wanted to ensure that the next time there was a leadership crisis, I would not be viewed as the only viable option to provide interim leadership. I must say, though, that I enjoyed serving as interim president, and I appreciate the board having named me president the month before the new president took office. It was a nice gesture of appreciation for my service and assured that I would go down in history as the fourth president of the MSM.

During my tenure, to achieve our leadership development goal the Leadership Council, consisting of thirty-five institutional leaders, set aside four hours per month to discuss leadership. In addition to becoming familiar with one another, we shared mutual concerns. In a real sense, we became a team—a leadership team, which included vice presidents, deans, the directors of administrative offices, department chairs, and others.

Although I had been in several leadership roles in academia and government, I had never engaged in this type of leadership development activity before. It felt good, and we all grew as leaders. In June 2006, the Morehouse School of Medicine board voted to establish the leadership institute that bears my name, allowing me to continue my leadership development efforts. We were fortunate to receive funding from private and public sources, locally and nationally, to begin program development. We now have over $12 million in endowment, but the need is great.

The mission of SHLI/MSM supports the historic mission of Morehouse School of Medicine, which is dedicated to improving the health and well-being of individuals and communities; increasing the diversity in the leadership of health professionals and the scientific workforce, and addressing primary health care needs through programs in education, research, and service, with an emphasis on people of color and the underserved urban and rural populations in Georgia and the nation.

The institute's vision is to be a transformative force for global health equity. We value diversity, integrity, trustworthiness, consensus building, and prevention as priorities, and access to quality health care for all persons. Our long-term goals are to develop an ever-growing, diverse network of public health leaders in the United States and ultimately throughout the world, and to enhance the development of domestic and global health policies aimed at improving health and health equity, which add two significant dimensions to this effort.

Our leadership determined that three key components were required to create a sustainable, high-quality organization, and indeed they have proven critical to the institute's growth and success. The components are *endowment and long-term program funding, functional partnerships to help define and guide program growth over time, and a reputation for integrity and excellence.*

The institute's approach to developing global leaders includes sponsoring fellows and scholars who participate in an innovative curriculum, with a special emphasis on neglected issues, such as health policy development relative to disparities in health, mental health, sexual health, and family health. Programs are informed by an expert advisory board, well-qualified teachers who are experts in their fields, and community-wide mentors.

Since its inception, SHLI/MSM has worked to realize its mission and vision through three core leadership development programs and community-engaged and community-based projects.

The Health Policy Fellowship Program is a multidisciplinary ten-month postdoctoral program that utilizes community-based practicum learning. Professionals, public health leaders, and others focus on health policy and how to impact health policy. To date, seven classes of Health Policy fellows have graduated.

Fellows immerse themselves in some of the most important health policy issues of our times. The most recent class of fellows had the opportunity to study the Affordable Care Act while its legitimacy,[9] in states that had not agreed to extend Medicaid, was being considered by the Supreme Court. One week before the fellows graduated, the Supreme Court ruled in support of the ACA. The current political environment afforded the fellows an extremely rich experience.

The Community Health Leadership Development Program trains leaders from community-based organizations who are interested in advocating for health promotion and disease prevention in their communities. While initially focused on the metropolitan Atlanta area only, through a partnership with the CDC, the twelve-week program now engages leaders from nine states, whose travel and housing are supported by a grant from the CDC.

It is interesting that many pastors, when asked to refer members to the Community Health Leadership Program, referred themselves, and now, more than 30 pastors have completed the program. A total of 285 participants, including more than 40 elected officials (mayors, county commissioners, council members, state representatives), have completed the program. The program is in the process of assessing the impact these leaders have had on health promotion and disease prevention in their communities. We have recently received a foundation grant to put more focus on mayors in urban communities. We believe that this is a worthwhile endeavor because generally, in urban communities, mayors end up on the frontline of most crises, including health-related crises.

The Quality Parenting / Smart and Secure Children Parenting Leadership Program provides training to some 50 parents a year to improve parenting skills and thus enrich child development. Between 2012 and 2017, the program has graduated more than 305 parents of children ages 0 to 14. Focused on low-income African American families in high-risk neighborhoods, this program helps to enhance parents' ability to provide supportive, nurturing environments, ultimately fostering both improved physical and behavioral health outcomes for themselves and their young children. Initial impact measures for the program, which began almost four years ago, demonstrate a decrease in symptoms of depression among parents, and improvements in achievement of benchmarks in childhood behavior and learning.[10] We have also begun measuring the program's impact on breastfeeding and childhood obesity. As a result of the program's success, support was recently received from the National Institutes of Health (NIH) to replicate the program beyond Atlanta, to twelve states. This process has already begun in thirteen states, including Georgia.

The Introduction to Leadership Program is not intended to be a comprehensive leadership development program. It is an introduction to leadership and includes opportunities for medical students and others to spend one to two months learning about the problems of health disparities and the role of leadership in achieving the goal of health equity. It will, one hopes, be a source of motivation for participants to pursue service in this area.

Two other programs, which are now housed in SHLI/MSM, were both started before the establishment of the leadership institute and were later integrated into it. The Center of Excellence for Sexual Health was developed to implement actions proposed in the *Surgeon General's Call to Action to Promote Sexual Health and Responsible Sexual Behavior*,[11] with funding from the Ford Foundation. Its mission is to raise the level of national dialogue on human sexuality, and on sexual health and well-being. The inaugural class of the Community Leadership in Sexual Health Scholars Program began its ten-month training program in the fall of 2008. Two cohorts produced nine graduates (2008–2009 had five participants and 2009–2010 had four).

"Community Voices: Healthcare for the Underserved" was initiated with funding from the W. K. Kellogg Foundation. It has made tremendous strides in the development of research projects, implementation of program initiatives, convening of meetings and conferences, dissemination of publications, fostering leadership development, mentoring, community collaboration and establishing viable partnerships, and the execution of myriad strategies for informing health policy around oral health, juvenile justice, and prisoner reentry.

Leaders emerging from the leadership institute—some novices, others advanced—are diverse in race, ethnicity, gender, nationality, disability, and professional discipline. These leaders will focus on developing best practices, improving public health infrastructure, reducing health disparities, and promoting health equity.

The motto of the Satcher Health Leadership Institute at Morehouse School of Medicine is "Here, everybody teaches and everybody learns," and since we have learned from all of our students, we feel that our leadership development programs continue to grow in relevance and excellence. We believe that when leaders stop learning, they stop leading. SHLI/MSM encourages leaders to continue learning and to understand community resources that can help them do a better job of leading.

Finally, we believe that leadership at its best is mission-oriented. It is the mission that drives our programs and our decisions about the students, scholars, fellows, community leaders, and others selected to participate in our programs. The goal of eliminating disparities in health in the United States and achieving global health equity is one that resonates with us as our raison d'être. It was the mission of striving for and achieving health equity that motivated me from my near-death experience in Alabama, until this day, as I seek to help others become the best leaders they can be.

Chapter One

Lessons Learned from Fifty Years of Leadership

I N THIS CHAPTER I attempt to convey some of the important leadership lessons that I have learned during my long career in leadership roles, and before that, during my formative years. Events from my childhood, undergraduate college experience, professional training experience, and government service illustrate these lessons. To make them easily distinguishable, the lessons have been set in italics. I emphasize the importance of leadership as a team sport because leadership teams are crucial to the success and effectiveness of all leaders, and they are central to my approach to leadership.

Leadership lessons are learned by observing the behavior of other leaders as well as from one's own leadership experiences. My first and very important leadership lessons, before I became active as a leader myself, were learned from careful observation of other leaders.

18

For me, leadership lessons began on the forty-four-acre farm where I grew up, with seven siblings and parents who were serious about their responsibility to lead. Each of the children always had an assigned responsibility. Before I was old enough to work in the field, I had to carry water to my siblings who were working in the fields. That was clearly my responsibility, and I was expected to do it in a timely manner.

As a leader, it is important to understand one's responsibility and to communicate clearly to each member of the team his or her responsibilities. When responsibilities are assigned, they should be clearly communicated to all concerned and periodically inspected. Leaders should strive to be positive role models, for members of the leadership team and throughout an organization, in terms of trustworthiness, civility, and commitment to the community served.

As I got older, my responsibilities grew in terms of complexity and difficulty. I remember when I was responsible for feeding the chickens, then the cattle, then the mules, then milking the cow, chopping in the fields, and plowing the mules. Our parents monitored our work, and as my brother Robert liked to say, "They believe that you can't expect what you don't inspect"—and inspect they did. When the work was done well, they were generous with compliments and rewards. Through their own efforts, they modeled the qualities they expected of us.

Our parents also kept things in perspective. Neither of my parents finished elementary school, but for us, they made education a priority. They had not been many places—only once out of Alabama—until much later, as we children went to and graduated from college. They took special pride in our academic achievements. They also taught Sunday school, and my dad, who was a first-grade dropout, due to his father's problems with alcohol, learned to read with the help of my mom. He served as superintendent of the Sunday school for over twenty-five years. Our parents were positive role models.

From my parents I learned to clearly communicate expectations; carefully inspect the work done; give positive feedback when appropriate; and keep life in perspective for myself and those working with me.

In our home, teachers were held in high regard, and we were expected to treat them with respect. When we got into trouble in school and were punished, we did not report it to our parents because they saw teachers as heroes whom we were expected to obey— although some of my teachers had problems and perhaps did not deserve the respect that our parents thought they did. For example, I had a teacher who acted negatively toward dark-skinned children; she regularly required me to wash my hands. She said that dark skin was automatically "dirty skin." While this was never a pleasant experience for me, I managed to negotiate our differences while respecting her authority.

My dad articulated his general attitude toward the treatment of other people when he was telling me goodbye as I left for college. As I was preparing to board the Greyhound bus, to leave Anniston for Atlanta and Morehouse College, my father had these parting words for me: "David, I want you to promise me something," he said. I responded, "Yes, Dad, what's that?" He said that he knew that where I was going I would meet some people who would have more than me, and perhaps some who had less. "Promise me," he said, "that you will always treat everyone with respect." I promised him that I would, and until this day, in all of the positions I have held, and with all the people I have worked with, that advice has served me well.

I do not think any advice has been more important to me than that sage advice from Wilmer Satcher, who was wise in so many ways, and because of that he was a great father, a great man, and a great leader. I learned from him that leaders must treat other people with respect. It is not only right but also empowering to both parties, and it enriches the environment.

Morehouse College was the most important bridge in my history because it prepared me to go almost anywhere that I wanted to go thereafter. When I arrived at Morehouse, there were serious questions about my abilities. The Admissions Committee did not admit me until my chemistry teacher, Pappy Dunn, spoke with a Morehouse alumnus in Anniston about my performance. The committee said they had never heard of Calhoun County Training School, but they decided to take a chance on me. I left with great confidence. In addition to the quality of my education there, Morehouse provided an opportunity to observe quality and passionate leadership, especially from the president, Dr. Benjamin Elijah Mays, the civil rights movement's Dr. Martin Luther King Jr., and student leaders.

Dr. Mays spoke to the student body in chapel every Tuesday morning. Attendance at chapel was required every day except Saturday. When Dr. Mays spoke, we sat on the edge of our seats as he challenged and motivated us to "aim for the stars." But the quote that best reflects his tone was perhaps the one in which he said, "Whatever befalls your lot in life for you to do, strive to do it so well that no man living or dead or yet unborn could do it better." President Mays's personal commitment to excellence was apparent not just in his words, but in all that he did. He communicated it clearly and lived it constantly. He was deeply admired by all the students on campus and after they had become alumni, as well. He was admired for his integrity, his confidence, and his commitment to excellence.

In addition to the campus experience, this was also the period when Martin Luther King Jr. served as co-pastor of Ebenezer Baptist Church with his father, "Daddy King." As stated before, whenever my friends and I knew that Dr. King would be speaking, we would walk the five miles each way to hear him speak. He was the ultimate communicator in words and deeds. One of my favorite King quotes is: "We must somehow learn to live together as brothers and sisters, or we will all perish together as fools."

It is important for leaders to model the behavior we expect in those we lead. This is especially important when dealing with young people. First and foremost, leaders should set a tone of high expectations. Dr. Mays exhibited a commitment to inspect the behavior we expect in a very impressive fashion, as my parents did. When I went to Case Western Reserve University in the MD/PhD program, Dr. Mays would regularly write the dean inquiring about my performance. Fortunately, I got off to a great start, and Dr. Mays would often read the dean's letter to the Morehouse students in chapel as a way of motivating them and as a way of saying to them that Morehouse had done a great job of preparing me for the next step—and he was right. The dean of the medical school said he had never before received a letter from a college president about a former student's performance.

It is important for leaders to be effective communicators even if they are not outstanding public speakers. Leaders need to know how to educate, motivate, and mobilize, internally and externally. Jim Collins, in his book *Good to Great*,[1] points out that some of the most outstanding leaders were not charismatic speakers, but they were all great communicators.

I found participating in the civil rights movement as a student leader to be refreshing.[2] Following Dr. King and my upper-class leaders, such as Marian Wright Edelman (founder of the Children's Defense Fund) and Otis Moss Jr., I went to jail and prison at least five times. I was a serious student, but I could not pass up the opportunity to finally confront racism. The student sit-in movement afforded me that opportunity.[3] The confrontation with racism through that movement transformed me from victim to confronter to leader.

Once, along with four other students, I was arrested and sent to prison outside of Atlanta. We had been successful in fulfilling our goal to fill the jails, so when we were arrested, we were sent to prison.

A young white man who had been caught while spraying us, as if we were flies, was arrested along with us and sent to the same prison. Luckily we were released early when the John F. Kennedy presidential campaign asked the mayor of Atlanta to release Dr. King. He did release Dr. King, along with others arrested at the same time— including myself.

There were five students, and our leader was A. D. King, the younger brother of Dr. King. On the way to prison, A. D. had advised me to get rid of a knife I used to sharpen my pencils, since I usually studied in jail. I did not heed his advice because it was a very short knife (from my perspective), and its only purpose was to sharpen pencils. As we were getting ready to enter the prison, A. D. again asked all of us to get rid of anything that could be considered a weapon. Still not heeding his suggestion, as soon as we entered the prison, they discovered my knife and threatened to put me in "the hole." And even though A. D. King had advised me to get rid of the knife, he came to my rescue by pleading with the prison warden on my behalf. Thankfully, he was persuasive, and they put me in with the other students and prisoners.

When we were released, after the Kennedy call, A. D. King suggested that we should ask that the young white man, who had sprayed us with insecticide and been placed in a white area of the prison, also be released. At first we objected, but he convinced us that nonviolence was not just about refusing to be violent, but it was also about refusing to hate; it was about loving our enemies. When the young man was released and saw us, he hugged each of us, pledged that he would never again conduct himself in that way and that he would do everything he could to advance the cause for which we fought—our civil rights. While I learned that nonviolence is a powerful weapon for change, especially when there is clear communication, as demonstrated by Dr. King, I also learned the following valuable lesson about leadership: *Leaders must first man-age themselves, and self-awareness allows first for self-management, which empowers leaders to manage others.*

I would ultimately become head of the Atlanta student movement, which had been established by a group of Atlanta University Center students who formed the Committee on the Appeal for Human Rights.[4] I would also become president of the Morehouse College Student Government Association in my senior year. So I had many opportunities to lead, even as a student, and I had some great role models. I gained knowledge and confidence. But what led me to leadership roles was my commitment to equal justice.

When I went to jail, I took my books with me. Other students noticed that I stayed on the honor roll, even while going to jail, and frequently scored among the highest on examinations given after I had been released.

Younger students, who came through the Comparative Anatomy Laboratory, where I worked as a student laboratory assistant, noticed that I cared about them and made every effort to help them succeed. When the time came, students prevailed upon me to run for student body president because they already saw me as a leader, even though I had not yet held a leadership position. A leadership lesson that I learned early is that *leadership is not position dependent, but effective leadership often leads to positive positions of leadership. Caring is one of the most important qualities of leadership.*

Because of my experience growing up in Alabama, being a part of the student movement in Atlanta, and rising to a leadership role, I left Morehouse College for medical school with an attitude. My attitude was that *I was expected not only to become a doctor and practice medicine, but that I was expected to be a leader in medicine—a leader in the quest for health equity.*

When I left Atlanta and the South to attend medical school, African Americans were excluded from most medical schools in the

South, and most hospitals did not allow African American physicians to admit patients to their wards. I was on a mission, in many ways, to improve access and quality of care for those often left out. It was the passage of Medicaid and Medicare that forced most hospitals in the South to admit African American physicians and their patients,[5] in order to bill these federal programs. Just as the business leaders in Atlanta had decided that it was not in their best interest to continue excluding African Americans from their service or employment, hospitals in the South decided that they could not afford the risk of losing the finances that accompanied those programs.

My mission in medicine was clear to me long before I got to medical school. It started on that small farm in Alabama where I barely survived whooping cough and pneumonia, and where many children of color and in rural areas died of these infectious diseases. Then, my experience as a student in Atlanta convinced me that, against incredible odds, *I could confront racism, and I could help to change things*. Leaving for medical school, I believed that I had to help to change medicine and health care into more equitable ventures.

When one is clear about his or her mission, it is easier to decide what leadership positions or roles to consider and which to say yes or no to. It is important to have clear plans, and while plans will and should change, it is important to stay on course with the mission. *Leadership at its best, in my opinion, is mission-oriented*. The mission defines the journey, and the mission defines the goals and the energy with which we pursue them.

Today, students often come to see me to ask for advice. But it is amazing how often they come with the question, "How did you plan to become surgeon general?" They let me know they are interested in becoming surgeon general, even though some of them have not yet gotten into medical school or passed chemistry in undergraduate school. They are often disappointed when I tell them that I actually did not plan to become surgeon general, but, as with other leadership positions I have held, I responded to an opportunity. That opportunity was consistent with what I saw as my mission in life. I actually declined the first time I was offered the opportunity to be nominated for surgeon general. The position was never my goal; it was the opportunity to serve.

Although we are often tempted to be honored by positions of leadership, I have come to understand *that as a leader, it is not about me. Instead, it is about the mission served.* It is sometimes too easy for leaders to get carried away with themselves, especially if they are not adequately focused. *Mission-oriented leadership leads one to forget oneself and instead to get caught up in the institution's or organization's mission. Leaders must see their roles in leadership as bigger than themselves.*

Developing and managing the leadership team is a prerequisite for success. Not only should the leadership team be stronger than the individual leader, it should also be greater than the sum of its parts. But *in order for the team to function optimally, the team leader must be personally secure and able to motivate the team to greater heights.* The lesson learned is that *leadership at its best is also a team sport, and one of the most important responsibilities of leaders is to build, nurture, and manage the leadership team.*

When I was a third-year medical student and in the obstetric-gynecology rotation, I committed an apparent act of courage for which I have been praised and even honored. I was the only African American student in my class at the time. Because I was an MD/PhD student, my schedule did not allow much time for me to interact with the other medical students. On the first day of the obstetric-gynecology rotation at the University Hospital at Case Western Reserve, we nine students on the rotation were led into a room to learn the pelvic examination. At that time, before Medicaid had been fully implemented, patients who could not pay for their care were required to be subjects of the teaching program. On this particular day, there were four women (who happened all to be African Americans) waiting to be subjects of the pelvic exam by the students. We were in a line waiting to begin. I was immediately struck by the lack of privacy and dignity (there were no curtains) with which the women were treated. I refused to participate and walked out of the room.

The rotation director, who was shocked and angry, threatened to have me not only put out of the rotation but also out of medical school. I was later told that I was to see the dean the next morning, and I assumed that this would be the end of my medical school experience at Case Western. It was a turbulent night as I saw my whole future at risk despite all my hard work, including working in the laboratories and taking calls at night and while other students were away on vacation. After my second year on the MD/PhD program, I had married and was starting a family. My wife, Callie, recognized how disturbed I was about the upcoming meeting.

The next morning, I anxiously went to see the dean, Fred Robbins, who had won the Nobel Prize for his work in oral polio vaccine development. I thought that participating in the sit-in movements, being arrested, and going to jail were frightening, but this was the height of terror for me. Dean Robbins greeted me with a smile and complimented me on the quality of my work to that point in medical school; he recited the honors I had won and generally summarized my performance to date, as a prelude to what he was going to say to me. Dean Robbins said, "David, it seems that you've gotten yourself into trouble with the obstetrics and gynecology services." I acknowledged that I had and explained to him how I felt about the experience. Then he asked, "Do you know what happened this morning?" I didn't. He told me the other students had also walked out because they agreed with me that this was inhumane treatment of the women.

Instead of being put out of school, I became somewhat of a hero, especially to the nurses who had been concerned with the treatment of these women but were afraid to say anything. Later, at the request of the nurses but also as a way of attracting more minority students and residents, a special fund to support clerkship experiences for minority students was named for me. Case Western had come to believe, as I did, that diversity was enriching to the environment, and so they were beginning to invest in diversity. I was pleased to be associated with that effort.

Perhaps mine was an act of courage, but I now question if it was an act of good leadership. I think not, if you believe as I do now that *leadership is a team sport*. Even though I do not know what would have happened, I could have spoken with my classmates about the basis for my feelings and actions before I walked out, and assuming they would have joined me, there would have been far less risk to me. That remains a question in my mind.

If we believe that leadership is a team sport, then we must take every opportunity to build the team around us. Apparently, someone among the eight students I left behind took leadership responsibility and got the other students to walk out the next morning. I never found out who or even asked. In retrospect, I am indebted to that person and the other students. At any rate, and in spite of the limitation of this example, *leadership at its best is a team sport*. Throughout my career I have tried to remember that lesson.

Before going into government, I served as president of Meharry Medical College, in Nashville, Tennessee, for more than eleven years. In academia, the president has deans of schools and vice presidents for various areas. In our case, there were deans of the school of medicine, the school of dentistry, and of graduate studies. In addition, there were vice presidents for finance and business, institutional advancement, and academic affairs.

In some cases, a new president is able to adopt the existing leadership team and move forward, but as a rule, the new president puts in place his or her own leadership team. In my case, a combination of the existing and new members made up my leadership team. If the existing leadership members are unwilling to work with the new leader, toward a new vision or plan as appropriate, then the new president must act to shape a new team.

When I became president of Meharry Medical College in 1982, the institution was in a serious crisis, financially and academically. This crisis had been widely publicized, including in a major *New York Times* article, which predicted that the college would soon close.[6]

I chose to keep in place as executive vice president someone who had been at the institution for forty-plus years. Among other things, he had received the first NIH grant at Meharry and had very high academic standards. My own strategy for the college included prioritizing the development of strong academic programs, as a basis for overcoming debt and to support successful fund-raising. Before his death in 1998, C. W. Johnson wrote a book entitled *The Spirit of a Place Called Meharry* in which he wrote in great detail about our work together.[7] He was the nucleus of a leadership team during my years as president of Meharry Medical College. Johnson knew the school much better than I did, and together with my new vision, we were able to salvage Meharry's future.

I was, however, forced to make leadership changes, replacing some people who I felt could not buy into our new strategy or measure up to our expectations. *Our plans for academic renewal* became the nucleus of our program for moving the institution forward. It became the basis for our successful fund-raising campaign and for our recruitment of new faculty leaders. Obviously, we had to deal with the debt and general financial status, but our argument was that we had a plan consistent with our mission: The Plan for Academic Renewal. *Good leadership must have a plan and must be able to get others to buy into it.*

Plans are critical for any leader or institution. Individuals, foundations, and corporations like to know the plan to which they are contributing. But plans don't always work, and sometimes plans must change with new developments, new insights, and new opportunities. At such times, it is the mission that must keep the institution and the leader on track. Meharry had a very successful first phase of its plans for academic renewal, and we exceeded our fund-raising goal. We raised $38 million, or $5 million more than our $33 million goal. We brought in new academic leadership in all key departments and restored accreditations at every level.

The mission of an institution and its leader must be greater than the plan, which is put together to move the institution forward: the "why" of leadership is more important than the "how."

It became clear that Meharry could not survive or succeed without dealing with the basic problem of a lack of access to publicly funded facilities. Our major teaching facility, Meharry Hubbard Hospital, continued to lose funds in excess of $4–5 million a year. We gained access to Nashville General Hospital for students and teachers, which greatly enhanced our teaching experience. Unfortunately, we had little or no control over its operations but still carried much of its financial burden. And yet, given the mission of Meharry Medical College, publicly funded facilities that cared for the poor were critical to its survival and teaching facilities. For over 100 years, Meharry had been excluded from these publicly funded facilities, including not only Nashville General Hospital but also the Veterans Administration Hospital located on Vanderbilt University's campus. So in 1988, in a presentation to the Rotary Club in Nashville, of which I was a member, I introduced our proposal for the merger of the Meharry Hubbard and Nashville General Hospitals. This proposal, we argued, was consistent with our missions and critical to our survival. It was also in the best interest of the city of Nashville and its responsibility for the care of the poor. Meharry's mission was to assure access to quality care for the underserved like those served by Nashville General.

Together with the leadership team, leaders must take time to visualize the future and develop a plan that is consistent with that vision. However, *the vision must be bigger than the plan, and the plan must be open for input and modifications.*

The struggle to gain approval of the Nashville City Council went on for four years before the plan was approved in August of 1992. It included moving Nashville General Hospital from its present location to Meharry's campus while investing over $50 million to upgrade the Meharry Hubbard Hospital facility to become the Metropolitan General Hospital.

The struggle for approval of this proposal is detailed in *A Place Called Meharry.* The plans for Meharry Medical College evolved, but the mission remained intact and survived the most difficult period in Meharry's history. Leaders must take advantage of every opportunity to communicate their plan and the mission of the institution, and to communicate clearly and convincingly.

Both as the director of the Centers for Disease Control and Prevention and as surgeon general,[8] I was at a disadvantage in terms of the history I brought with me. I was the first CDC director with a background that did not include having worked at the CDC or in the Public Health Service (PHS). My background was in academia and in community leadership, including almost twelve years as president of Meharry Medical College. However, in putting together my leadership team at the CDC, I chose an outstanding public health scientist as my deputy director. Claire Broome, who was well known for her research, including having first helped to describe toxic shock syndrome,[9] was highly regarded at the CDC and throughout the Public Health Service. No woman had ever been deputy director of the CDC or even head of an institute or center at the CDC.

When I chose her as my deputy, she was in her eighth month of pregnancy; the deck seemed to be stacked against her. She turned out to be the best choice.

Claire Broome provided me with the inside knowledge of the CDC and public health services that I needed when dealing with any issue. She was the core of my very strong leadership team and my liaison to the rest of a well-functioning leadership team. I brought new and innovative strategies for reaching communities that had not been reached by the PHS before. We partnered with community organizations.

Childhood immunization levels, by the age of two, were just over 50 percent nationally in 1993. When I began work at the CDC, the rate in Vermont was 70 percent overall, but in Detroit only 29 percent. Part of our strategy was to engage the National Council of Black Churches in our efforts; it paid off. We were able, with President Clinton's leadership, to get Congress to remove the financial barriers to childhood immunization, and we brought new technology to bear to better inform physicians of the immunization status of children they saw in their offices. We were able to raise the immunization rate *to over 80 percent by 1996*, and to virtually eliminate disparities in childhood immunization.

To be effective, the leadership team must be diverse, and greater than the sum of its parts, and certainly greater than the top leader alone. Leaders who are comfortable with themselves are *eager to have people on the team who know much more about certain areas than they themselves know, thus greatly enriching the leadership*.

We were a strong and well-balanced CDC leadership team, including the appointment of the first ever associate director for Behavioral Health, Dr. Marjorie Spears. Recently, I was invited to return to the CDC to speak at the twentieth anniversary of the Behavioral and Social Sciences Working Group.[10] There are now over four hundred members of the Working Group and they have made a tremendous contribution to CDC programs, including HIV/AIDS and chronic disease control. Mrs. Rosalynn Carter still considers this one of my major contributions as director of the CDC.

I served as CDC director from October 1993 to February 1998. At that time I became the first CDC director to be appointed United States surgeon general. I also became only the second person to serve simultaneously as surgeon general and assistant secretary for health. The first was Dr. Julius Richmond, who served under President Jimmy Carter and started the very important Healthy People Program,[11] in which goals and measurable objectives for each decade were set for the health of the American people.

In addition to the responsibility of communicating health messages directly to the American people (e.g., the Surgeon General's Reports), the surgeon general oversees a six-thousand-member Commission Corps. This corps is virtually on call seven days a week, twenty-four hours a day to respond to any emergency threatening the health of the American people, such as the September 11, 2001, World Trade Center attack in New York City and the anthrax outbreak experience during my tenure.

I was at a disadvantage in that I had not previously served in the Commission Corps. My appointment carried the rank of four-star admiral since I had served as both surgeon general and assistant secretary for health. Again, the real challenge was putting together a quality *leadership team*. The two most critical appointments would be those of deputy surgeon general and principal deputy assistant secretary for health.

The clear choice for deputy surgeon general was Vice Admiral Kenneth Moritsugu, who had been in the Public Health Service and the Commissioned Corps for more than thirty years. I met him when I worked at the King/Drew Medical Center in Los Angeles, where he was the head of Region IX of the PHS. In 1976, he had been helpful in our efforts to begin a residency program in family medicine at King-Drew. Moritsugu proved to be a great choice. I came to rely upon him to virtually run the office as I traveled throughout the world speaking about the Surgeon General's Reports, as well as the Surgeon General's Prescription.[12] We released the first ever Surgeon General's Report on mental health,[13] the first ever report on oral health,[14] and the first ever report on overweight and obesity.[15] We had a great team with great communication. *Leadership is a team sport, and ultimately the team and how it functions is critical.*

For my principal deputy assistant secretary for health, I chose Dr. Nicole Lurie, who was a professor of public health at the University of Minnesota. She was a leader in public health and an outstanding academician who had demonstrated an unusual commitment to making public health relevant to the needs of the public. We also had two outstanding deputy assistant secretaries for Health, Dr. Virginia Betts, a nurse psychologist, and Dr. Beverly Malone, also a psychologist and former president of the American Nurses Association. I believe it was perhaps one of the strongest and most productive leadership teams ever assembled in the Public Health Service (PHS) and the Commissioned Corps.

When I left after four years, Drs. Moritsugu and Lurie stayed on. Dr. Moritsugu would serve as deputy surgeon general for two more surgeons general and as acting surgeon general on two occasions. Dr. Betts later became commissioner of Mental Health for the state of Tennessee and Dr. Malone was chosen by Prime Minister Tony Blair to head the nursing service for all of Great Britain. She served there for six years before returning to the United States as CEO of the National League for Nursing.

In short, I have been blessed with outstanding leadership teams in my career, especially during my government service. To the extent that I have been successful, I owe it to the quality of the leadership team and other lessons learned along the way.

Chapter Two

From Health Disparities to Global Health Equity

H EALTH DISPARITIES are preventable differences in *the burden of disease, injury, and violence,* or in opportunities to achieve optimal health experienced by socially disadvantaged racial, ethnic, and other population groups and communities.[1] These disparities are unjust, unfair, and *directly related to the historical and current unequal distribution of social, political, economic, and environmental advantages.*

The Centers for Disease Control and Prevention, the National Institutes of Health,[2] and several other agencies have defined "disparities in health." Common to most definitions is a focus on real differences in health-related outcomes between different groups of people (not only different racial and ethnic groups), including sexual minorities, people with disabilities, people with mental health disorders, people who live in rural areas, and others. These differences are generally considered preventable.

When the Institute of Medicine published its 2002 report on health disparities, *Unequal Treatment: Confronting Racial and Ethnic Disparities in HealthCare*,[3] the focus was on differences in health care services, quality of care, and access to care. The report documented these differences in groups labeled "Majorities and Minorities." In the early 1940s, when I had my near-death experience with whooping cough and pneumonia, issues of access to health care and quality of care were both paramount, but they were also related to racial segregation, discrimination, and poverty.

More than fifty years later, as surgeon general and assistant secretary for health, I bore a major responsibility for the health of the American people and for leading in the development of goals and objectives for the Healthy People 2010 Initiative.[4] As mentioned in chapter 1, the Healthy People Initiative was begun in 1979,[5] during the administration of President Jimmy Carter, by Surgeon General Julius Richmond, with the vision of making America's communities healthier and happier places to live. This program articulates broad goals, objectives, and inputs for the health of the country for the next decade. It is important to note that *Healthy People 2000*,[6] released in 1990, spoke to disparities in health with a commitment to *reducing* health disparities but not *eliminating* them.

Healthy People 2010 was released in January 2000 and introduced the commitment to eliminate disparities in health.[7] The overarching goals were to increase the quality and years of healthy life for all Americans and to eliminate racial and ethnic health disparities. The commitment to eliminate disparities (not simply reduce them) galvanized the public health community by making the goal more measurable and by demonstrating a level of boldness that had not been verbalized before. Goals are aspirations, and these aspirations push everyone concerned to work for high achievement. Goals do not, in and of themselves, have timelines, but they allow for objectives that establish timelines for components of the goals.

As a result of the commitment to eliminate disparities in health, Congress passed the Minority Health and Health Disparities Research and Education Act,[8] which led to the creation of the National Center for Minority Health and Health Disparities (NCMHD) at the NIH, in 2000. The center was renamed the National Institute on Minority Health and Health Disparities (NIMHD) in 2010, with authority for grant making. At the CDC, the articulation of the new goal led to the development of the Racial and Ethnic Approaches to Community Health Program (REACH).[9] The REACH program funded communities directly to develop programs geared toward the elimination of disparities—for example, programs that would address quality of care and control of conditions such as hypertension and diabetes.

That particular day in Washington, DC, when *Healthy People 2010* was to be released, was a very unusual day. Six inches of snow covered the ground and continued to fall when I went out for my morning walk on the NIH campus. Even though the federal government was technically closed, Secretary of Health and Human Services Donna Shalala and I agreed, by phone, that we should proceed with the release, given all the preparation that had taken place, especially since more than two thousand people were waiting in hotels, having traveled to Washington to participate in the ceremonies. Among those gathered were the ministers of health from both Egypt and Uruguay, to whom I had made a commitment to attend the release of *Healthy People Egypt* and *Healthy People Uruguay* later that year.

There is no substitute for well-defined goals and their associated objectives. Setting goals and objectives forces us to make clear decisions and to associate them with measurable outcomes and even timelines. Perhaps even more important, goals and objectives allow us to come together in our commitment to progress. Such was the nature of our gathering.

It is important to make clear the reality and nature of disparities in health. We can measure the frequency of occurrences of various diseases, measure mortality rates, and compare them among different groups. In the United States, among others, there are significant disparities in infant mortality, cardiovascular deaths, excess deaths, cancer prevalence, and the occurrence and complications of diabetes. While there has been great improvement in health for both African Americans and Caucasians, especially in areas such as infant mortality, cardiovascular disease, HIV/AIDS, and even cancer mortality, the ratios between African Americans and Caucasians have not improved. For example, African American infant mortality rates remain 2.4 times the white rates.[10]

What if we were equal? After leaving government and moving to Morehouse School of Medicine, I participated in a study, published in the *Journal of Health Affairs* in 2005, that asked that question.[11] In an attempt to find an answer, differences in mortality rates between Caucasians and African Americans were measured and compared, using data from 1960 through 2000. These mortality rates included conditions such as cardiovascular disease, diabetes, HIV/AIDS, and cancer, but we also looked at issues related to access to care and measures such as the level of insurance coverage. We calculated that if we had reduced mortality ratios such that by the end of the twentieth century we would have eliminated disparities in health, the picture of health for African Americans would be quite different. For example, in the year 2000 there would have been 83,500 fewer African American deaths, including 24,000 fewer deaths from cardiovascular disease; 22,000 fewer from diabetes; 7,000 fewer from HIV/AIDS; and 4,700 fewer from infant mortality or death during the first year of life.

These so called "excess deaths" were the targets of efforts to reduce and ultimately eliminate disparities in health. However, our concerns were not limited to mortality. If we had eliminated disparities in the uninsured, or the risk of African Americans being uninsured, so that African Americans had the same insurance coverage as whites, in the year 2000 there would have been 2.5 million more insured African Americans, including 620,000 more insured children. Such measures of disparities will allow us to measure our progress toward health equity as we move forward.

It should be noted that African Americans and Caucasians are the only two groups in the country for which these kinds of reliable data exist. In fact, there are data going back to the turn of the twentieth century, when overall life expectancy in this country was forty-seven years—forty-nine for whites and thirty-four for blacks.[12]

In addition, the study compared mortality ratios for blacks and whites by sex and race, from 1960 through 2000. Changes in these mortality ratios over this period included a positive shift for African American females compared to African American males and Caucasians. In retrospect, these changes reflected some major changes in the social environment, including education, drug use, and incarceration. In each of these areas, African American males had been adversely affected.

In the 1980s, the downward trends for African American males were dramatic, corresponding to the introduction of crack cocaine and the subsequent increase in crime, including homicide, leading to a dramatic rise in incarceration.[13] By the end of this period, increases in attendance and graduation from college by African American females corresponded to an increase in school dropouts and incarceration for black males.[14]

Disparities, however, are not hopeless conditions, because we can improve health care and health outcomes through better access and quality of care. We can measure quality and reward desired behaviors as well as improve health behavior. Finally, we can change the negative social conditions into which people are born, grow, learn, work, and age. We now know that social determinants of

health (SDH), such as education, income, and safety, have a tremendous impact on health outcomes.[15] The CDC now uses this type
of information in pursuing its strategies for reducing the spread of
diseases, such as HIV/AIDS and tuberculosis.

In the early 1990s, former CDC Director William Foege and Mi-
chael McGinnis, head of the Office of Public Health Science, published an article in *JAMA* on the determinants of health.[16] They
concluded that the four major determinants of health were individual biology/genetics, health care quality and access, environment,
and behavior. In examining these four determinants, they found that
health care accounted for only 10–15 percent of the variation in
health outcomes; individual biology/genetics accounted for 20–25
percent; and environment, 20–25 percent. Behavior accounted for
40–50 percent of the variations.

While I was director of the CDC, these observations of the importance of behavior led to the 1996 release of the first Surgeon
General's Report on the importance of physical activity and nutrition.[17] I would later release the Surgeon General's Prescription for
physical activity, nutrition, the avoidance of toxins, responsible sexual behavior, and management of stress.[18] It would make a huge impact if all people would adopt these health behaviors, but social
determinants actually influence behavior. For instance, people living and working in underserved communities often do not have
safe places to be physically active or easy access to fresh fruits and
vegetables. The very people with the most to gain have the hardest
time making these changes.

In 2004, after I had left government and returned to the Morehouse School of Medicine, where I was serving as president, I was
asked by Director General J. W. Lee, of the World Health Organization, to join the Commission on Social Determinants of Health
(CSDH).[15] I had previously worked with Director General Lee when
I was director of the CDC, and he was heading the infectious dis-

ease unit of WHO. I served on the commission from 2005 to 2009. The commission traveled to diverse countries throughout the world to assess how health was being impacted by changes in social determinants of health (SDH) and how those changes might impact health outcomes. Among countries visited by the commission were Kenya, Canada, Brazil, Chile, China, Japan, and Australia. We also visited New Orleans, Louisiana, wanting to understand the impact of a natural disaster such as Hurricane Katrina on the health of the people.

The commission defined social determinants as "the conditions in which people are born, grow, develop, learn, work, and age."[15] We were particularly interested in how these conditions affected health outcomes. For example, we saw how certain countries had targeted child development by intervening to improve the social conditions of children, including providing daycare from the age of three months and later integrating it with education and healthy living. We saw other examples, in which countries had not targeted the social determinants of health. These included Nairobi, Kenya, where we found one of the largest slums in the world.[19] Notably, Kenya was considering investing heavily in building a major hospital but had not found the means to provide running water in the slum. This was in the midst of a high rate of school dropouts and an increase in HIV/AIDS. We encouraged them to make investments in running water and education the priorities to improve health.

Perhaps it is relevant to this discussion that the CSDH first resisted scheduling a visit to the United States as a part of the information-gathering process, even though there were three Americans serving on the commission: Dr. Bill Foege, Dr. Gail Wilensky, and me. This reluctance to visit the United States, I think, was related to the fact that the administration of President George W. Bush was not supportive of our work, financially or philosophically. Since Dr. Foege and I had both been nominated to our federal roles by a Democratic administration, we thought that the Bush administration might be more supportive of the CSDH if a Republican appointee could be added. So, early in the process, the commission chose Dr. Wilensky, former head of the Healthcare Finance Administration under the first President Bush. This move did not garner more support from the Bush administration, but Dr. Wilensky brought great expertise in areas that dealt with financial policy, so she was a tremendous addition.

Members of the commission also did not see the United States as relevant to its work, given the country's relative wealth, and the reality that, in spite of its wealth, the United States had and continues to have major health disparities. They saw this as a profound lack of commitment to the health of all its citizens. Having worked to help rebuild the health infrastructure in New Orleans after Hurricane Katrina,[20] the commission was convinced that examining the differential impact of disaster on communities and ethnic groups in New Orleans would help to inform its report on the social determinants of health and would impact the goal of global health equity. The commission's visit to New Orleans was funded by three private foundations, but it received no support from the federal government. It reminded me, again, of the importance of private foundations.

Our visit to New Orleans in late 2008 included tours of the hardest hit areas, particularly the low-income minority community of the Ninth Ward. We interacted with survivors of the hurricane, with surrounding communities, and with the mayor and other local officials. That post-Katrina visit was deemed one of our most important trips. Clearly, a major disaster can undermine the social health infrastructure of a community, and it certainly did so in New Orleans.

The visit to New Orleans made clear that disparities in health impacted the experience of citizens before, during, and after the hurricane. When the levees broke, because of their low elevation, communities in the Ninth Ward suffered the greatest onslaught.

This predominately African American community was also the least likely to have transportation. Thirty percent of its residents did not own cars,[20] which could have helped them to evacuate the area of the hurricane and subsequent flooding. Those who caught the bus to the Superdome, or traveled to Memphis, Atlanta, or Houston, in most cases would not have the means to return or rebuild after the hurricane. There was also not much for them to return to. Of those who couldn't evacuate, almost two thousand people, disproportionately black and poor, died. It was helpful that I had been asked earlier by the NIH and HHS to work on rebuilding New Orleans' health infrastructure.

After Hurricane Katrina, there was an increase in uncontrolled diabetes, hypertension, and a dramatic increase in depression. From 10 to 20 percent of the people screened positive for depression,[21] in both New Orleans and Baton Rouge. Together, we (the NIH's National Institute for Minority Health and Health Disparities) prioritized the rebuilding and reopening of the major hospitals for the poor in New Orleans. When Charity Hospital was replaced by University Medical Center New Orleans as the main trauma and safety net hospital, it included tributaries that reached out into the community to provide primary care and early access.

Our visit to New Orleans helped to solidify our appreciation of the role of social determinants of health and their impact on health outcomes, even in the face of a natural disaster like Hurricane Katrina. The commission found that these conditions were also shaped by the distribution of money and resources at the global, national, and local levels. And finally, we found that changes in SDH often require policy changes related to health insurance coverage, the environment, and access to healthy lifestyles.

I must also point out that there is significant interaction among these various determinants, such that access to health care, if it involves caring and committed physicians, may result in dramatic improvements in behavior, as well as in the environment, which could be seen in the reduction of lead levels or other measures. But negative environments make it difficult to attract quality health care providers, and thus, health care is itself a social determinant of health.

Measurable outcomes may lead to a resetting of goals. These measurable outcomes constitute a form of evidence that strategies are working or not working. When we fail to measure the outcome of our efforts, we do harm to our vision.

In January 2009, WHO released the official report of the CSDH, *Closing the Gap in a Generation: Health Equity through Action on the Social Determinants of Health*.[15] This report had a major impact on *Healthy People 2020*,[22] which was released in 2010. Whereas *Healthy People 2010*, released in 2000,[7] included two very important goals— increasing the years and quality of healthy lives and the elimination of disparities in health—the *Healthy People 2020* goals represent the incorporation of the recommendations of the commission and the goal of health equity. The four overarching goals of *Healthy People 2020* are:

- To attain high-quality, longer lives free of preventable disease, disability, injury, and premature death;
- To achieve health equity, eliminate disparities, and improve the health of all groups;
- To create social and physical environments that promote good health for all; and
- To promote quality of life, healthy development, and healthy behaviors across all life stages.

These goals have moved us to a new level in the effort to eliminate disparities in health. This focus on the environment, social relationships, income, and education represents new targets for the Healthy People Initiative.

If health equity involves the conditions, especially the social conditions, in which people are born, live, learn, work, and age, then our efforts must be focused on creating the opportunity for people to achieve optimal conditions for good health, whether those conditions be related to education, income, environment, or safety.

So the journey from the goal of eliminating disparities in health, as articulated in *Healthy People 2010*, to the goal of health equity, articulated first by WHO in 2009 and incorporated into *Healthy People 2020*, is a journey that the Commission on Social Determinants of Health helped to define in its four years of global travel.

This journey will require vigorous leadership and recognition that policies related to health and the social determinants of health must be amended. We need to develop integrated leadership to promote an attack on disparities in health, by attacking the social determinants of health, including the public health system itself.

The Affordable Care Act,[23] passed during the Obama administration, represented some major policy changes. These changes greatly impacted access to care, reducing the uninsured population by over 20 million people. The ACA also made mental health an essential health service, requiring parity of access for the first time in the United States. The Mental Health Parity and Addiction Equity Act had already greatly impacted access,[24] but the ACA put in place the policies that could be used to make sure these measures were implemented. This meant that provider coverage and services had to include mental health; these were indeed essential health services.

The ACA allowed for children to stay on their parents' insurance policy until age twenty-six, and perhaps most notably, *the ACA made it illegal to exclude anyone from coverage due to any preexisting conditions!* This was very important for so many families, in which children may have a mental health problem, diabetes, a disability, or something else that would prevent them from accessing the insurance market. Today, with a new administration under President

Trump, the Affordable Care Act is threatened. But the passage of the law, and the failure of the many efforts to repeal it, show that we have built momentum in the fight for health equity. The journey continues and, in my opinion, cannot be easily stopped.

Chapter Three

When Leadership Confronts Failure

L ET US ACKNOWLEDGE at the onset that it is easier to remember and to discuss our successes than our failures. Yet, the lessons that we can learn from our failures are just as important as the lessons we learn from our successes, if not more so. The ability to accept our failures, and deal with them, is one of the most important roles of leadership.

While a personal failure on the part of a leader may not be an institutional failure, an institutional failure is almost always a failure of leadership. As with individuals, sometimes institutions fail because the nature of the attempt was flawed. By correcting the flawed attempt, we become better than we thought we were.

Learning from failure can move us to even higher levels of success. In 1976, when I became interim dean and CEO at the Charles R. Drew University of Medicine and Science,[1] in Los Angeles, the stakes were quite high. The founding dean, Dr. Mitchell Spelman, had given up on the Drew mission to bring quality health care to the Watts community from an academic medical center that trained doctors who would then stay on to practice in that community.

It is not altogether clear that the department chairs and other leaders believed that I could succeed, or if they were pushing me into the path of an oncoming truck. But I believed in the mission of the institution, and I loved the Watts community, in which I had become quite involved, including developing, founding, and operating a free clinic in the basement of Second Baptist Church. The stakes were indeed high, and success would certainly establish me as playing a leading role in medicine and public health, but I took on the role because I was committed to the mission. Fortunately, we were able to work out the Drew–University of California Los Angeles (UCLA) partnership. As a public university that was challenged to serve all the people, UCLA needed more black students. The partnership with Drew provided more black students, even though those students would spend their last two years in Watts, in keeping with Drew's mission.

When the Board of Regents of the University of California approved the merger of Drew and UCLA on May 28, 1978, it was a major accomplishment. Shortly afterward, a family crisis led me to return to Atlanta, but Drew was on its way, and my former mentor, M. Alfred Haynes, returned to lead its redevelopment. I will always feel good about what happened at Drew, and the institution it became. To succeed in the face of failure is one of the great joys of leadership. Likewise, failure is one of the great pains of leadership.

In the meantime, Meharry Medical College in Nashville was facing another crisis, perhaps its greatest. It had graduated almost half of the black physicians and dentists in the country, and most of them had gone on to practice in underserved rural and inner-city communities.[2] It was, however, being choked by an ever-increasing debt on the Meharry Hubbard Hospital, which provided care to a very poor and underserved community. The debt was already in excess of $20 million and growing rapidly, as Meharry cared for patients who were poor and many not eligible for Medicaid. When the *New York Times* came out with the major story, projecting that Meharry Medical College would soon close,[3] the country took notice.

At the time, one of the members of Meharry's presidential search committee was a Meharry alumnus named Ezra Davidson, with whom I had worked on the sickle cell research project at King-Drew, where he was chair of the Ob/Gyn Department. From his role in my selection as the interim dean at Drew, he apparently argued that if anyone could lead Meharry Medical College from its strapped present to a better future, I should be able to do so.

Soon the invitation came for me to come to Meharry for an interview. I immediately declined, but I began to receive calls asking me to at least come for an interview. One of those calls came from Dr. Henry Foster, chair of Ob/Gyn at Meharry, whom I would later tap to serve as vice president for Health Affairs. Needless to say, the effects of the closure of Meharry Medical College would be colossal, and almost no one wanted that to happen. Although its survival would be a major accomplishment, the risk of failure was very high. Although I did not want to be president, I cared deeply about Meharry Medical College and its mission, and so I agreed to go for the interview without thinking that it would go any further. During the visit, I came to realize just how important the institution was. By the time I left I had decided that I actually had nothing more important to do than to take on this high-stakes challenge, if selected. In retrospect, it is difficult to explain why I believed that we could succeed at Meharry. I deeply believed that Meharry was right in its mission and that it deserved to survive. Some might say that failure was not an option, but it was.

Many considered the institution on the brink of failure, but we were successful in stabilizing the college and implementing the plan for academic renewal. This included a five-year fund-raising campaign, with the goal of raising $33 million and selecting new leadership for many departments. We approached President Ronald Reagan and Congress to forgive the long-term debt, arguing that Meharry had more than repaid it, given the service Meharry provided to the poor in Nashville.

We had not stopped the financial drain resulting from the care of patients who could not pay for their care, so, even though we succeeded in our fund-raising campaign and in getting forgiveness of the long-term debt, Meharry's burdens were still heavy. Although we had gained access to participate in residency training at Nashville General Hospital, we still received no reimbursement for patient care since Vanderbilt University still held that contract, as it did with the Veterans Administration Hospital, which was located on its campus. This holdover from the days of segregation in the South had not been significantly challenged.

The college's future depended on a genuine partnership, and the use of publicly funded facilities in Nashville, with Vanderbilt University Medical Center. Recognizing this, in 1988, at a meeting of the Nashville Rotary Club, of which I was now a member, I presented our proposal for the merger of Nashville General Hospital and Meharry Hubbard Hospital. Since Nashville General Hospital was crumbling and would cost hundreds of millions of dollars to rebuild, we felt that merging the hospitals, using the fairly new Meharry Hubbard Hospital, was the logical solution. We felt it was in the best interest of care, as well as in the financial interest of the community. Meharry Hubbard Hospital was also located in North Nashville, where most of Nashville's poor lived, and its long-term debt had recently been forgiven.

I had been president of Meharry for over six years and was fairly well-connected in the community and the city, and I was determined to fight for this proposal. I had a broad base of relationships and had spent many hours discussing the proposal with Dr. Ike Robinson, the vice president for Health Affairs at Vanderbilt University, trying to get Vanderbilt to join us in the proposal. Vanderbilt refused, but vice president Robinson promised that he would not speak out against the proposal. And he did not. But I knew that Vanderbilt's support on the hospital board, which would ultimately make the decision, was strong. Thus, the presentation of the proposal at the Rotary was the beginning of an almost four-year debate. We were able to engage the community and the City Council in that debate. In February 1992, the hospital board voted to reject the proposal before it could get to the Nashville City Council. It was a split vote, I believe five to three against the proposal. This was a major setback for us at Meharry Medical College. We had given much time and enormous energy in support of the proposal, and now it seemed the proposal was dead. We could see no other viable options. We had failed in our most important effort.

The Meharry Medical College board meeting was coming up, and for the first time, they would confront me as a failed president. Despite our efforts, I would face them empty-handed in terms of a plan for Meharry's future. It was a terrible feeling, compounded by the fact that my dad had recently died, adding tremendously to my burdens. My dad had suffered from chronic lymphocytic leukemia for several years and succumbed to it after much suffering, including the amputation of one of his legs.

For the 1992 commencement, Dr. Al Haynes, my old friend and mentor, came from Los Angeles on the same flight as a couple of Meharry board members. He was to receive an honorary degree. When he arrived, he invited me to come to his hotel room for lunch. He was deeply troubled and concerned that, on the flight, he had overheard one of the Meharry board members brag that they were going to Nashville to "fire a president." He wanted me to be prepared for a very difficult board meeting. Ever since the hospital board's negative vote, I had had trouble sleeping. I would generally wake up before three in the morning and could not go back to sleep. Failure is a terrible burden for a leader to bear, especially when so much is at stake. Even worse, I had no alternative strategy to present to our board.

After the discussion with my friend and mentor, I knew what I had to do: I needed to leave and allow the institution to move on. When it came time for me to meet with the board, I asked for a closed session. Facing a board that might be considering firing you definitely merits a closed session. I apologized for our failure to get the vote of the hospital board for this hard-fought proposal. I asked them for something that I had never requested in my sixteen years of academia experience. I needed an eight-month sabbatical to get myself together. During that time, I would understand if the board decided to recruit a new president. I would be prepared for that.

The Meharry Medical College Board of Trustees refused to respond immediately to my proposal, wanting to discuss it among themselves. They thanked me for my proposal and for taking responsibility for our failure. The next day we came back together after they had deliberated. They reminded me of all that I had been through over the previous few years, including my dad's death. They did not support my going on sabbatical. They wanted me to take a short break, and they were prepared to support my continued leadership as being in the best interest of the institution. In essence, they were saying, "David, this is your ball. We need you to take it to the end zone."

Needless to say, I was rejuvenated and eager to move forward. I made an appointment with the mayor of Nashville, Bill Boner, who, though a friend of our institution, had been hands-off with the proposal; he was also a Vanderbilt graduate. First, he chastised me for not coming to see him sooner. Then we talked strategy. He wanted to hear again the major points of our proposal. In response, he felt that our best argument was the financial one, that by accepting our proposed merger, the city would benefit financially while continuing to provide quality care for the patients in a fairly new facility.

However, the mayor wanted us to present our proposal to a group of financial experts and leaders that he would put together. Among others, it would include the founder of Shoney's Restaurant, the head of Hospital Corporations of America, and the head of the Sunday School Publishing Board. Mayor Boner promised that if this group agreed with us about the financial impact of our proposal, he would ask the Board of Hospitals to reconsider and support a proposal to the City Council for the hospital merger. To make a long story short, the special committee found that the merger would have a very positive financial impact on Nashville and that in our proposal we had underestimated the potential impact.

Armed with this report, Mayor Boner took the proposal back to the hospital board, which then voted to proceed with it, and by a vote of five to two, passed it on to the City Council. The City Council voted overwhelmingly to support it, and in August 1992, our proposal passed the City Council. It was a great day for Meharry, it was a great for me, and I think it was a great day for the City of Nashville. In many ways, it was a new day for all of us.

In retrospect, the most important decision I made was not to in any way challenge Meharry's Board of Trustees. Even though I believe that they had come to fire me, I don't think that any institution can survive unless the clear authority of the board is respected. Whenever that authority breaks down or is in question, the future of the institution is in jeopardy. I don't believe that any institution can survive without a clear chain of command, beginning with its board of trustees. In the absence of a board, authority must be clearly established and followed. If I had taken on the board, I would have had the support of the faculty, the students, and many in the community, but I would have weakened Meharry as an institution. My having taken responsibility for the failure of our proposal liberated me and gained the board's support—a lesson that I will never forget. In fact, following the meeting, the board was more supportive than before.

Less than a year after the City Council had approved the merger, I presented to the board a proposal to launch the largest fund-raising campaign in Meharry's history—a $100 million campaign. Between 1982 and 1986, as a part of a plan for academic renewal, we had set a goal to raise $33 million, and we had actually raised $38 million. We felt that we now had the momentum to succeed in a $100 million campaign. The chair of the board, Dr. Frank Royal, and his wife, Pam, asked to meet with me in their hotel room that evening. They gave me a check for $25,000 as a lead gift; we were on our way, and I was deeply encouraged.

Our plan was to begin by identifying 100 Meharry alumni who could contribute $100,000 each, or $10 million, as a "Lead Alumni Campaign." We wanted the alumni themselves to lead this campaign. The alumni component of the campaign was very successful, and when I left Meharry the next year to become director of the CDC, 85 of the 100 identified alumni had already made their commitment, and we were ahead of schedule. The next year, an alumnus contrib-uted $1.6 million, the largest alumni gift in Meharry's history. But it was how we dealt with a major failure that led to this success.

Looking back on this experience more than twenty-five years later, leadership lessons abound. One of the most important and challenging issues facing leaders, especially in a business or an in-stitution, is the relationship between the leader and the board of trustees. That is being played out today at many historically black colleges and universities (HBCUs). Failure of a major institutional effort is invariably and appropriately seen as failure of the leader. Although boards have ultimate authority, the most important role of the board is to hire and fire a president.

An institution cannot survive with a dysfunctional board. When external bodies, such as accrediting agencies, feel that a board of trustees is in disarray, they target the institution and its accreditation and/or its viability. Strong boards sometimes have to make decisions about their own leadership in order to correct their performance. If called upon, the president may play a role in this discussion, but it is the responsibility of the board.

In interpreting my relationship with Meharry's Board of Trustees, regarding the failure of our proposal for the hospital merger, I offered them the opportunity to let me go. Their refusal to accept my quasi-resignation (eight-month sabbatical) was, I believe, based on their belief that I could lead the institution out of a historically difficult situation. They asked me to stay on and continue to lead our struggle, without any threat or condition, but made it clear they believed that I could be successful. As a result, we came out of the negative vote much stronger as a team and moved on to a significant victory with the second Hospital vote. Failure can be devastating; it is painful and penetrating; but most leaders experience failure along the way. How it is handled is critical.

When I was rejected for admission to Duke University Medical School in 1963, I felt as if the world had ended. I had worked hard and excelled in college at Morehouse, while leading the student sit-in movement and the student government my senior year.[4] I had many sleepless nights during my final months at Morehouse. But I continued to lead and to pursue the unknown world ahead. That road led me to the Case Western Reserve School of Medicine and its MD/PhD program. It was that program that put me in a position to truly lead in medicine and in public health for years to come. I was also able to win an NIH fellowship, which provided the funds for my tuition, as well as my room and board.

How leaders handle failure is a real test. We can gain tremendously from watching others lead through failure and come out rejuvenated and stronger than before. Televangelist Dr. Robert H. Schuller reminded us that success is never-ending and failure is never final, unless we let it engulf us and stifle our spirit.[5]

While I have taken on several high-level positions, I don't necessarily recommend it. Leadership can take place from many different levels or positions, not just high positions. Leadership lessons are often best learned before one is in a high position. Sometimes high risk is associated with our values, benefits, and beliefs, and we are able to rise with the challenge that comes with failure. However, when we fail, the way we fail is what matters most, and next is our response to that failure. It is tempting to run away from failure and leave it behind. But it is only by enduring our failure and learning from it that we are able to come out of it stronger than before. By asking ourselves, What could I have done differently? What could I have done better? we are able to both avoid failure and respond appropriately to it the next time. Leaders must exhibit hope and confidence, especially in the face of failure and disappointment. Our vision must allow us to see beyond failure and to see it as temporary.

John Heyward was right, in 1546, when he said, "There are none so blind as those who will not see."[6] My dad, Wilmer Satcher, did not finish any grade in school, but he had a lot to teach me nonetheless. Early in my tenure at Case Western Reserve, I ran into hard times. I was working at night and on weekends, being on call to conduct laboratory tests when patients came into the emergency room after the lab had closed. It was impacting both my sleep and study, and I still could not see how I could earn enough money to pay room and board, and part of tuition going forward. Fortunately, I got a few days break to go home during the Christmas season. There I unloaded my fears and the burdens that I was facing to my parents. I remember my dad's words as we sat around the fireplace. He said, "I have no doubt that you're going to make it. You'll find a way, and when you do, having worked so hard, it will mean much more to you than if it had been easy; you will do much more with it." He urged me to embrace the struggle, and with a vision of a brighter day. My dad was a person of deep faith, and so am I. His words reminded me that I had survived because of their faith and mine.

Two months later, my research advisor, Dr. Neal McIntyre, and I submitted my research proposal to the National Institutes of Health because Dr. McIntyre felt it was unusually good and that the NIH might support it. Indeed, the NIH did fund my research proposal. Their funding included enough for tuition and room and board. It was an amazing day, and I remember calling home to tell my parents. Again, my brush with failure was a springboard to something better; because I had saved money, not anticipating NIH funding, I was able to help my parents get running water in our home, for the first time, in 1964.

Without an education, my parents were great parents and great leaders in the community and in the church. They lived their lives under the hammer of segregation and discrimination, but they never lost their vision of a better day for themselves, and especially for their children. We were taught to have unwavering faith in God's grace in the face of hardship, discouragement, and potential and actual failure. I believe that, in part, my attraction to difficult leadership roles—especially, when I believe deeply in a mission—is related to my upbringing and the way I have witnessed and experienced the ability to overcome difficulties and difficult times. My parents believed deeply in God and loved their children and their neighbors, and so do I. And that faith is the major force in my life.

For those of us who dare to lead, particularly in difficult situations, sooner or later our leadership will be put to the test. It will be put on the line, and when leadership is put on the line, it is both an opportunity and a challenge to which leaders must respond. There's a dramatic difference between individual success and leading a group or an institution to success, but they both depend on communicating our vision and confidence. Supporting those who walk with us, or fail us through difficult times, is a special challenge and a special opportunity. They become stronger and so do we.

Coordinating the efforts of a team of leaders is also a special challenge, which portends greater accomplishment. This is when leadership is clearly a team sport, when a team functions with mutual confidence, tenacity, and support. Together the team achieves what no individual can do alone. Together the leadership team reaches what individual leaders cannot, and together the leadership team has courage and perseverance that a single leader cannot have—but it all begins with leadership.

Sometimes leaders set the bar high for what they want to accomplish during their tenure. In the case of Meharry Medical College, where the crisis was immediate and the institutional need was so great, there was no choice but to set the bar high and to plan for the long term. In some ways, that increased the opportunity for failure and the impact of success. While looking back on my rejection by the Duke University School of Medicine is no longer as painful, it still reminds me that failure can be painful but indeed is never final. Doing well in biochemistry after coming out of jail is an example of setting a more modest goal when faced with great odds.

So, what is the optimal time for a leader to leave a leadership position? Obviously, in the face of major failure, the leader will almost always need to leave, to give the institution the best chance of moving forward with new leadership. But I believe that after achieving a major goal is also a good time for transition. It defines the leader's tenure as successful and also enables the institution to attract strong leadership for the future.

I provided a signal to the Meharry Medical College Board of Trustees that would have made it easy to fire me after the failure of our proposal for the merger of the Meharry Hubbard Hospital and

Nashville General Hospital. But I still harbored some optimism, and I was relieved when the board did not ask me to resign. I still think that it was important that I made the offer to resign in the face of this apparent failure. In fact, I was newly energized by the board's expression of support for me to get back into the struggle to solve the institution's historic problem. Before the board's decision, I felt alone in my failure, but the board's decision said, We are in this together and we believe in your leadership. After the success of the follow-up proposal and the successful beginning of a major fund-raising campaign, I settled in for a pleasant tenure as Meharry Medical College president. For the first time since becoming president, I did not feel the pressure of crisis.

Then I heard that the Department of Health and Human Services was seeking new leadership for the Centers for Disease Control and Prevention and that I had been highly recommended—having done well in Watts, in Los Angeles, and in Nashville—as someone who could succeed in bringing public health protection, such as childhood immunization, to some of America's hardest to reach communities. I saw this as another of the kind of challenge I have always found attractive. But I was now comfortable as president of Meharry, and I felt no pressure as I interviewed for the CDC position.

Meharry Medical College had become comfortable, but the CDC position was clearly my kind of challenge and the reason why I went into medicine and public health in the first place. Failure may be a good time to leave an institution, but success that can be passed on to the new leader, in my opinion, is the ideal time to leave. So again I walked away from my comfort zone to assume a new position of high risk and challenge. Whenever failure is clearly a risk, but success carries great promise for national and global impact, I tend to be attracted. When aiming high, the risk of failure is with us, but the fruits of success can be irresistible.

Chapter Four

The Need for Clear Communication

L EADERS MUST BE ABLE to communicate clearly, both internally and externally; it is one of the most important responsibilities of leadership. Of course, this does not mean that all leaders must be great orators, but it does mean that they must be able to effectively relate to their followers, the organizations' missions, goals, and programs, as well as specific strategies and plans. Indeed, not all leaders are outstanding public speakers, but all leaders need a communication strategy that assures the thorough and timely transmission of key information for action.

One of my favorite stories is the one about the new surgeon general who was getting rave reviews everywhere he spoke, and he was really feeling good about himself—so much so that he asked his support staff if they could take him somewhere where people would otherwise not get a chance to see him or hear him speak. They decided to take him to a nursing home.

At the entrance, they were greeted by a lady in a wheelchair, who was greeting everyone. It was not her job to do this; she just did it because she enjoyed doing it. Upon encountering her he asked, "Ma'am, do you know who I am?" She did not respond, so he asked her again. Finally, she said, "I don't know who you are, but if you go to the front desk they will tell you who you are." Audiences tend to remember stories of this kind, and appreciate their impact on the environment created by the speaker. Such stories help to enhance the relationship between the audience and the speaker, and sometimes, years after I have given a speech, I run into members of the audience who remember a story I told to make a point, even though they may not always remember the point.

Years after leaving the position of director of the Centers for Disease Control and Prevention, I was asked to return and be keynote speaker for its celebration of the birthday of Dr. Martin Luther King Jr. In attempting to describe his special strengths as a speaker, I said that, more than anyone I had known or heard, Dr. King had the ability to educate, motivate, and mobilize. He shared valuable information; he gave his audiences hope and determination; and he often moved his audiences to action—whether for the Montgomery bus boycott or the student sit-in movement,[1,2] which often resulted in students going to jail. Even people such as my parents, who had less than an elementary school education, could understand what he was saying and were often moved in their spirit and in their action.

Dr. King was also a minister, and I heard him speak on many occasions. He was very well educated and often used what we call "big words." However, his explanations of difficult concepts from the Bible and from philosophy brought them to life for our times. He effectively shared his knowledge, experiences, and yes, his dream. In the process, he brought audiences from where they were to where they needed to be. Dr. King not only connected with his audiences, but he moved them to a new level of hope and determination.

Not all leaders need to be as articulate as Martin Luther King Jr. was, but a common element among good leaders is the ability to communicate clearly about problems or concerns and about how to address them. Good leaders must be willing and able to share information with their target groups and with the public. In short, the best communication educates, motivates, and mobilizes the target group.

Because of the importance of communication, the media can be a valuable ally, especially for the underdog. This was demonstrated in Birmingham, Alabama, when a very powerful and forceful police chief, Bull Connor,[3] called out dogs on children and adults who were demonstrating with Dr. King. For the first time, the media showed televised pictures of this event to people across America and the world. The impact of these photos led to the passage of the Civil Rights Act,[4] and to a great extent, the Voting Rights Act.[5] Many people said they watched in disbelief, unable to believe that "this was happening in America," and they came to see it as not just a Southern problem but an American problem—which needed changing.

Leaders are often respected for what they know, but they are remembered and followed for what they share. They must be committed to sharing ideas, plans, needs, hopes, and dreams, and their written and spoken words must be consistent. Written words generally outlast spoken words. In order to communicate effectively, those in charge must know and be comfortable with their mission and the contents of their message. Speakers must know their audiences in order to have an impact on them.

Ernest Hemingway said, "I like to listen. I have learned a great deal from listening carefully. Most people never listen."[6] The most underutilized form of communication is listening. Listening may be active, passive, aggressive, or creative.

Active listening has been defined as "mindfully hearing and attempting to comprehend the meaning of words spoken by another in a conversation or speech."[7] In passive listening,[8] communicators are using their ears to observe without giving any feedback or asking any questions; just listening. Sometimes, we need to listen passively. It takes patience to listen, not just to hear what is said, but to reflect on it, or in some cases, just to enjoy it. Proper listening can be therapeutic, especially for a leader caught up in the struggle of day-to-day work. When we listen, we not only promote ourselves and our own understanding but also build understanding and confidence among those we lead. Both active and passive listening build teams and community. When we listen to others, especially those who serve under us, we send the message that we respect them and value them enough to give them our time and attention and to work with them in finding the best path ahead.

Creative listening is finding a way to get followers to share what they might not otherwise share.[9] Sometimes it begins by sharing just enough with the audience to start a meaningful discussion. Here we are seeking input to our own thinking or reflection about an issue. At other times, we might merely present the topic at hand, putting it into perspective, and then listening for a response. As physicians, we have been taught to create the kind of environment where our patients feel comfortable sharing with us things they ordinarily would not share with others. Our job is to make the patient feel safe before asking potentially difficult or embarrassing questions. It is one of the things that I like best about medicine, because I know that most people need someone they respect and trust to listen to them.

For physicians and others, it is sometimes the nature of the questions asked; sometimes it is the way they are asked. There's an old quote in medicine: "People don't care how much you know, until they know how much you care."[10] This is certainly true of the doctor-patient relationship, as it is of other relationships, as well.

Finally, aggressive listening solicits and elicits information from those with whom we work.[11] It is on the other end of passive listening and may include elements of creative listening. Sometimes it is done by provoking a response. Sometimes it is framing the issue so that it provokes a response. Certainly our family hour at Meharry Medical College and director's hour at the CDC were meant to stimulate discussions around an issue of importance to the nation and the agency.[12] But in almost all cases, listening requires an element of patience. It should be based on concern for the issue(s) and for the persons involved or engaged. The gift that I tried to give the staff at Meharry and the CDC was my time and attention. They knew that I respected them enough and cared enough to share myself with them.

Whether listening is active, passive, creative, aggressive, or sometimes a mixture of two, three, or all four, listening is a critical part of effective communication and thus effective leadership. Recognizing the importance of listening also reflects a level of self-confidence that is free of the need to impress others.

For many years now, the favorite part of my presentations has been the question-and-answer period at the end. That is because I often get feedback that informs me about my delivery and sometimes helps me to understand the audience better. It is always interesting to me that some people are so obsessed with the need to impress the speaker or audience that they have trouble getting their questions out. And there are those who use the Q&A period to grandstand for the rest of the audience. Nevertheless, this is communication, and it builds community and mutual respect for all participants.

Effective leaders should not feel the need to convince audiences that they have all the answers or that they must give definitive answers for every question raised. Instead, leaders must sometimes commend the questioner or audience for the quality and relevance of the questions, some of which the leader may have not thought about before. Here, the leader exemplifies a commitment to learning and to personal and organizational growth.

Some leaders communicate best in one-on-one situations—a very personal setting. Others communicate best in small group meetings, for example, with a leadership team or in a classroom. Still other leaders are at their best when communicating before large audiences.

I believe the best leaders are able to balance these different settings and communicate well in all three. In a strange way, I am more comfortable speaking before large audiences than in one-on-one or small group settings, even though I have grown in each area over the years. I believe I have a form of shyness that leads me to be less comfortable in a small group than with larger audiences, which are less personal. In order to grow in these areas, one must acknowledge weaknesses and want to overcome them, and it is important to point out that it is practice that moves us toward perfection.

My public speaking began when I was a child speaking in church, where I got a lot of positive feedback. (My dad, as a deacon, spoke quite well before a church congregation.) Later, public speaking was a required course at Morehouse College, one that we took very seriously. And my college president, Dr. Benjamin Elijah Mays, was certainly a great orator.[13]

Dr. Martin Luther King Jr. is best known for his "I Have a Dream" speech,[14] delivered at the 1963 March on Washington.[15] I helped to plan the march while a student leader at Morehouse College, but I was unable to participate in it because it took place in the first week of my first year of medical school in Ohio. I also remember many of the short quotes Dr. King weaved into speeches and sermons. One such quote is, "Life's most persistent and urgent question is, 'What are you doing for others?'"[16] Another is, "Darkness cannot drive out darkness; only light can do that. Hate cannot drive out hate; only love can do that."[17] This is the kind of quote that both captures one's attention and motivates one for the work ahead.

Rosa Parks expressed the feeling that led her to resist. She said that she was just tired, and had made up her mind not to give up her seat to a white man again. There is nothing so powerful as a made-up mind.

I am convinced that just as important as the words in a speech is the passion with which a speech is delivered. That was certainly true of Dr. Mays, Dr. King, and my father. The message must not only be heard but also felt in order to educate, motivate, and certainly to mobilize.

It is interesting that not all good teachers are good speakers. My public speaking professor at Morehouse College was not himself a great public speaker. When he spoke in chapel, he seemed awkward and out of place. But in the classroom he drove his points home quite well and thereby helped many students develop superior speaking skills.

Communication does not work unless there is bilateral access. The environment of an organization is often shaped by the extent to which such bilateral communication takes place.[18] In part, it can be expedited by the leadership team, which places people who are on the team close to the people who may be further away from the top leader. The leadership team works best when its members listen to those below them and communicate their concerns and ideas to the leader and the rest of the team as is appropriate.

Ideally, however, it is best when information and concerns can be communicated directly to the leader. One example is during a family hour, or director's hour, which I describe in chapter 5. But that setting does not always work when the issues are sensitive. Here, the open-door strategy can be helpful. The leader can set aside one hour or more per week when individuals may schedule a walk-in for five minutes or so to share ideas or concerns, or just to introduce themselves to the leader. There are pros and cons to this approach, but my experience is that it has a positive effect upon the environment. This was especially true with students in the dental school, as illustrated below.

As president of a health professional school where women were historically underrepresented, I was once told that women in one of the schools were being taken advantage of—threatened by faculty if they did not comply with sexual advances. I was not convinced that the female students were entirely comfortable coming to see me with their concerns about this, so I designated a reliable female administrative assistant to hear their concerns. She was a mature community-leader type and a mother of three children, including a daughter. I then announced that students could schedule brief meetings with this assistant to discuss anything that they were not comfortable discussing with me. I was later told that this strategy had worked quite well. In fact, according to the students, the announcement alone virtually eliminated the problem. It was unusual for a president to even discuss these issues, so the announcement was probably initially quite impactful. It sent a message that I was determined to protect female students from exploitation and determined that they would have access to communicate their concerns to me. Sometimes, the mere act of providing access and communication, especially for sensitive issues, is enough.

The arrangement sends two kinds of message: first, it said that we cared enough about the issues to make a special effort to deal with them; second, it said that we as an institution would not tolerate an environment of gender or sexual exploitation. The same message is important when the issue is race, racism, ethnicity, or sexual orientation or preference.

After forty years of history, Morehouse School of Medicine has its first female president and dean. There are many things about her that I admire, but foremost is her commitment to open com-

munication. She engaged the entire institution in a strategic planning process over a two-year period, with quarterly town-hall meetings for input and feedback. The plan has a mission statement and
goals and a succinct vision statement—"leading the creation and
advancement of health equity."

Everyone at the institution is expected to remember and be able
to recite the vision statement, be they students, faculty, staff, or
administrators. It is important to be able to share your values and
goals so clearly and succinctly. This strategic plan has served to
expedite communication and fund-raising, and all that we do as an
institution. There is indeed no substitute for clear communication,
and more and more, institutions are moving in the direction of more
open communication with their entire population.

Communication and access to open communication can be the
solution to several kinds of problems. An environment that encourages listening is probably the most important aspect of communication. Clear communication must take various forms. At its
best, it expedites good relationships and productive teamwork. One
might say that clear communication helps to develop productive
relationships; but by the same token, good relationships expedite
communication.

Chapter Five

The Need for Continual Learning

P RESIDENT JOHN F. KENNEDY SAID, "Leadership and learning are indispensable to each other."[1] Leaders must be committed to continuous learning and must create an environment where people are rewarded not only for the answers they have but also for posing important questions—the answers to which move their organizations forward.

Certainly, the challenges facing leaders are dynamic, and leaders cannot be static in their response to these challenges. If leaders fail to keep learning, they will be unable to keep pace with the requirements of their mission or the people they are leading. Leaders who stop seeking learning opportunities often find that they are no longer relevant to the leadership needs of their organizations.

Effective leaders must continually learn about themselves. They should ask the following questions: What kind of leadership team will I need to be successful? What are my major weaknesses and strengths? Who are the people to best complement my work to move this organization forward?

Every leader has weaknesses that can negatively impact the advancement of the institutional mission. Since leadership is a team sport, those who surround and complement the leader are critical to the organization's success. A strong leadership team, with the leader at the hub, is greater than the sum of its parts. In knowing themselves, leaders are able to select team members who will best complement them.

Sometimes leaders learn more about themselves while they are struggling to lead. Leadership itself is a learning experience, and dealing with internal and external expectations can provide many lessons. When I was appointed director of the Centers for Disease Control and Prevention,[2] I was the first director to come from outside the organization, and it was important for me to be clear about what I could do and what I expected others to do.

Leaders must learn to deal with disappointments and keep moving forward. Not all plans work out, but all plans have the ability to teach us lessons. Leaders cannot afford to dwell on those things that did not succeed. Instead, they must look for the lessons in those failures. In addition, they must not be afraid to ask why, in the face of failure or success. Leaders must learn from those they serve by focusing on their assets as well as their deficits. When faced with new challenges and encounters, leaders must not miss learning opportunities.

The leadership team is very important to ensure effective functioning of the organization. Once the members are in place, leaders must continue to learn more about the team, in order to optimize its use. Interaction with the leadership team on a regular basis is an important learning exercise, as well as a part of the strategic action plan.

Although I was the leader among Atlanta University Center (the largest consortium of African American Institutions of higher education) students during my senior year, it was a Spelman College student who suggested that we go on a hunger strike when we were arrested for trying to buy food in a restaurant. I was skeptical at first but agreed. That idea and the global publicity that resulted led the Atlanta business community to end segregation.

As a student leader during the student sit-in movement, we did not have an office or a budget. We had no computers or cell phones, but we communicated effectively with each other, even if it meant walking to meet or leaving phone messages or sharing notes.

Some team members might already be in place when the leader arrives, and in many cases some will be asked to stay. Those existing team members who fit the needs of the new leader can be a valuable asset to the organization and its leader, but the relationship must be dynamic, and it must continue to grow. My working relationship with the vice president at Meharry Medical College, Dr. C. W. Johnson,[3] who was already in place, was an example of that kind of relationship. Together, we developed the plan for academic renewal, and he came into his own as never before, after having spent fifty years at Meharry. Articulating the challenges facing Meharry and planning for academic renewal appealed to Dr. Johnson, who had been the first Meharry faculty member to receive a competitive NIH grant.[4] He immediately got on board with the plan and became a major factor in our success. Clearly, I learned at Meharry that being the leader did not mean that I knew the most about the issues. I learned to use the knowledge of other team members.

Similarly, there must be continual growth by leadership team members brought on by the new leader, in their relationship with the leader and the overall team. This can only happen if the commitment to continual learning starts at the top. As new goals are set and new strategies defined, a learning team is able to rise to whatever challenges present themselves.

Each year, each month, each day brings new challenges and

new opportunities. As president of Meharry Medical College in the 1980s, I was responsible for a dynamic student body. Every year a group of students completed their learning and graduated, and I enjoyed handing the students their degrees. It was one of my great pleasures. Every year, a new group of students in medicine, dentistry, and graduate studies joined us at the institution. At least four years separated them from the students who graduated that year. In short, in many ways they came from a different world than their predecessors, and so we had to try and understand the world from which they came. We had to be continual learners. Likewise, our graduates were entering a dynamic world as new alumni; they would have different needs and expectations from the world and from the institution. We needed their support, and they needed us.

A large percentage of our students depended on loans and left school with large personal debts, averaging around $150,000. This was especially true since our students came from families who were less likely to be able to make large financial contributions to their schooling. On the one hand, we looked to our alumni for contributions to the school, but on the other hand, we needed them to pay off their debt to the federal government so that we could continue the program for new students who needed to borrow.

On one occasion, the federal loan program threatened to withhold loans from our student loan program if our alumni did not remain current in their debt payment.[5] Without the student loan program, most of our students could not have paid tuition, and we could not have paid our institutional bills. We were in a difficult position, so we made a difficult decision: we threatened to take our alumni to court if they did not repay their loans. It seemed a terrible thing to have to do, but we had to protect our current students and their access to student loans. Fortunately, our alumni responded, and their rate of loan repayments began to increase, saving the student loan program for our current students. It was a problem that

we had never experienced, and we met the challenge to come together as administrators, faculty, alumni, and students in order to
save our programs, which we did.

It was quite an eye-opening experience for all of us. It was certainly a major communications challenge. New problems require
new thinking on the part of all involved, and if leadership fails the
learning test, so will the institution. Had we done a better job of
educating and motivating our students to appreciate the critical importance of the loan repayment program while they were still students, we could have prevented or reduced delinquencies in loan
repayments. As we did a better job, our alumni did likewise.

The Vaccines for Children Program at the CDC was intended to
increase the percentage of children immunized by two years of age
from 55 percent overall to 80 percent.[6] It required us to enhance
our technology to help physicians know where a child was on the
immunization schedule. It also required us to find new partnerships in the community and to share information. Certain black
church organizations had to learn the importance of the campaign
and what they could do to contribute to it. Together we all learned
how to move forward toward a strategy for promoting the health
of our children. We did, and childhood immunization rates in the
country rose from 55 percent by the age of two, to 80 percent,[7] with
most disparities eliminated. It was our ability to learn that kept us
moving forward, and we are still learning.

Leaders must also continue to learn about the people they serve
and from the people they serve. As premed students at Morehouse
College, everyone agreed that the greatest challenge was in courses
like chemistry and physics. The chapters were sometimes difficult
to read, and it was not always easy to maintain concentration. Someone along the way recommended that we go to the end of the chapter, and try to answer the questions and solve the problems before
we read the chapter. I took this advice and became quite commit-

ted to this approach through undergraduate college, medical, and graduate schools. It was a great way to learn, and one that I continue to recommend. Become familiar with the questions and/or the problems before reading the chapter, and look for the answers as you read. Getting a clear understanding of the problems helps one to focus and concentrate.

This approach to studying and learning has made a major difference for me. In my junior year at Morehouse, a professor from Lockheed Aircraft Company came to the Atlanta University Center to teach physics to all of the undergraduate students who needed to take it.[8] Physics was a course that almost everyone regretted having to take, but it was a virtual requirement for medical school admission. The professor was somewhat doubtful of our ability to learn such difficult material, and the class showed not only deference, but fear of him and the subject.

One day he started by referring us to the questions/problems at the end of the chapter. He asked the students to share any questions or concerns that they felt they would have in solving the problems. One of the students selected a very difficult problem and asked the teacher to help solve it. The professor started to demonstrate how he would solve the problem. However, he got to a certain point and seemed confused; he started over but got stalled at the same point. I had solved the problem as part of my study the night before, so I raised my hand and volunteered that I might be able to solve the problem. He said, "Be my guest," and handed me the chalk. I went to the blackboard and without much sophistication, I worked through the problem as I had done the night before. The professor was astounded. He had no idea that any student in his class could solve a problem that he had trouble solving. From that day forward, the professor treated me and my classmates with a special kind of respect, and so did the assistants who taught the laboratory component. Fifty years later, people who were in that class still tell this story, and I am grateful to the person who gave me this valuable study tip.

Now, I knew that I was not so smart; I had just focused on identifying difficult questions and problems as a studying strategy. The same method was useful during my year as interim dean and CEO at Drew University of Medicine and Science in Watts. Because I knew that the major challenge facing the institution was getting its undergraduate medical education program started, we decided to target this issue.

In order to start our medical education program, we would have to partner with UCLA, since UCLA already had the faculty, classrooms, and laboratories for the two-year basic science curriculum, which were the first two years for medical school. Both institutions had some discomfort about working together, and I had several discussions with the dean at UCLA, Sherman Mellinkoff,[9] who was the longest-serving dean in the country. However, equal concern and doubt existed in the Drew School and its supporting community. I had to work both sides of the track in trying to get our medical education program going: that was my goal. Dean Mellinkoff could not get to know and become comfortable with the community served by Martin Luther King Hospital, but he was willing to get to know me, and become comfortable with me, and use this as a basis for supporting the proposal. In that sense, we were successful in our communication.

In West Los Angeles, where UCLA is located, Watts was viewed as a place of poverty and violence (e.g., the Watts riots). Drew was committed to working to bring public health and health care to that area. Many on the Westside were skeptical. On one occasion, an outstanding black physician in the Drew community challenged me to a radio debate about our partnering with UCLA, about which he had serious doubts. I accepted his challenge because I thought it was an issue that needed to be discussed in the community. It was a lively one-hour debate in which I tried to drive home the point that we needed to move forward with our medical school plan, and we needed the UCLA partnership in order to do it. Dr. Hill continued questioning the trustworthiness of UCLA working in the Watts community. It was not clear who "won" the debate, but I decided to commend him as if he had won. He was quite moved that I gave him the "victory," and it endeared him to me from that day forward, while I felt that I lost nothing in the process.

Yes, the debate and my assessment of it opened the door to an ongoing relationship. Soon, this physician became a major supporter of my leadership, and with his help we were able to move forward with the Drew-UCLA agreement. In May 1978, it was approved by the Board of Regents of the University of California. By not accepting the view of many, that I had won the debate, I was after all winning something more important—the respect and support of Dr. Hill and his community of supporters. Sacrificing short-term victories can often be important for long-term success. Certainly, Dr. Hill's contribution to our effort at the King/Drew Medical Center was much more important than what may have been considered a victory in the debate. It was a lesson I will never forget.

The analogy to leadership and learning, I think, is that leaders do not have to pretend to have all of the answers. Leaders must, however, be committed to learning and to identifying, for themselves and others, the most difficult problems and questions. Leaders are never too old to learn, and we all both teach and learn from one another. We must not seek to thrive in the comfort zone of our own expertise.

At the Satcher Health Leadership Institute we acknowledge that our students have more than needs or deficiencies; they also have assets and resources. Their backgrounds, history, or concerns are different from ours in many cases, but if we are to serve them successfully, we must know more about them. This can only happen if we give them the opportunity and permission to teach or share with us from their areas of knowledge or expertise—ones that society often does not acknowledge. When they realize that we value what they have to offer and want to learn from them, they become better students and share more fully in the classroom or in the community, wherever they might be. They also are less hesitant to ask questions and are not embarrassed to admit the things they need to learn.

The fellows at the leadership institute, who do their practicums in agencies such as the CDC and CARE International,[10] have taught us about barriers that can significantly hamper their access to learning experiences with those agencies. For example, we have worked with the CDC to remove or lower barriers in the area of increased security following September 11, 2001. To the extent that the CDC is comfortable with us and the screening that we do when admitting or selecting fellows, the less rigorous they seem to be with our fellows.

Although the Community Health Leadership Program began with a focus on local students, we made it a national program when a broader group expressed their desire to participate but needed support for travel and housing to spend the time necessary to meet the requirements of the program. Because of our students, we also developed a modified curriculum, whose objectives can be achieved with a consolidated one- to two-week curriculum, rather than one day a week for twelve weeks. By adapting to the needs of a broader base of students geographically, we have been able to modify our teaching and learning program.

Students in the quality parenting, or Smart and Secure Children's Program, taught us that our concern for developing children needed to expand to concern about parents and their needs as well. Because of them, we no longer limit our evaluation and monitoring to the children. We also measure the impact of the program on parents' risk for depression and other related disorders.

Leaders must have the courage to act. Doing nothing to advance our mission or to overcome a crisis is not acceptable. However, action often leads to mistakes. We must learn from our own errors and also from those that other leaders make.

In analyzing leadership mistakes it is important to ask ourselves the following critical questions:

- Why did we decide to do what we did?
- Were our actions adequately thought out and planned?
- Did we have adequate input into the decision to act?
- Was our timing correct, or should we have waited before acting?
- Did we have the right team in place, and what did we lose from our mistake in terms of time, money, and other resources?
- What did we gain from our mistakes, and where do we go from here?
- How do we get to where we want to go from here?

Leaders must also learn from their successes. It is important to stop and ask, What did we do right that we should preserve as we approach other problems? What did we learn about each other that could be useful and even vital for future successes? We tend to debate how important it is to stop and celebrate our successes. We should take inspiration from our own achievements, but I also think it is essential to stop and assess our successes in terms of the lessons learned and the implications for the future.

We must learn to know and appreciate the resources available to us. In what I often called the battle of Nashville, which resulted in the merger of Meharry Hubbard Hospital and Nashville General Hospital, and perhaps saved Meharry Medical College from impending demise, we learned to know and appreciate our resources internally and externally. We started the monthly family hour at Meharry Medical College early in the hospital board's consideration of the merger proposal. We used it to share information about the status of our effort to get the board to approve the proposal, Our monthly family hour meetings resulted in much broader appreciation of our team. For example, some of our employees, armed with better knowledge of our strategic goals, took it upon themselves to educate their churches and their neighborhoods, and to get people out to City Council meetings to support our cause when the council was considering our proposal.

Many of these people had been at Meharry all along, carrying out their day-to-day responsibilities, but armed with a new level of knowledge and motivation, they became leaders in their areas and communities. In short, we had resources that we did not know we had until we opened up to our "broader team." It was a tremendous lesson for me.

Finally, leaders must continue to learn about the mission for which they serve. Leaders must not take their mission for granted. Every goal carries different meanings and implications for different people. It's necessary for a leader at any level to remain aware and adaptable as understanding of the mission evolves.

Chapter Six

A Three-Dimensional Perspective on Leadership

B ASED ON THE OPPORTUNITIES I have had to work with leaders in their various capacities, I am convinced that there are several important qualities that effective leaders should possess. First, I think that leaders should care about the missions of their institutions and the people they serve. As such, leaders are always learning—about the mission, about themselves; and about those they lead. Effective leaders are decisive and willing to take responsibility for their decisions; they have the courage of their convictions and are willing to act on those convictions. To do this, leaders must have confidence in themselves and be able to inspire confidence in others. Thus, good leaders have the ability to motivate and inspire others to act. Leaders should be willing to take risks if the potential benefits are important to the mission of the institution. They need to be problem-oriented and creative in their approaches to solving problems. Leaders are team builders. And finally, leaders should respond to opportunities, challenges, and crises in ways consistent with their values and the best interests of the institution or organizations they serve.

I have observed leadership from a three-dimensional perspective: (a) observing those whom I have followed, (b) experiencing leadership from a personal perspective, and (c) helping others to develop leadership skills.

As a child growing up, I came to appreciate my parents' caring and commitment to their family, always working to assure that their children would have opportunities they did not have. Their mission was clear and their dedication to it was impressive. Also, as I observed my dad as a deacon in the church and in his role as superintendent of Sunday school, I was impressed that, even though he lacked education beyond the first grade and possessed a limited vocabulary, he often made things clear by telling memorable stories, many of them with a humorous edge.

I would later use the art of storytelling as I worked to help people understand the mission of Meharry Medical College or the Morehouse School of Medicine. While serving as president of Meharry, I noticed that President Ronald Reagan was a master at storytelling. I attended a State dinner in the Rose Garden at the White House in the mid-1980s, where President Reagan told the Meharry story, as I sat at the table with him, the president of Costa Rica, and others. President Reagan chose to tell the story of Meharry,[1] as opposed to giving statistics about its operation and the nature of its relationship with the federal government. In so doing, he was both entertaining and enlightening. Likewise, Dean Sherman Mellinkoff, the long-serving dean at UCLA, in the 1970s would often use storytelling with a humorous touch to keep our discussions positive when they were on the verge of becoming negative or heated.

Once when we were having a discussion about missions—University of California Los Angeles vs. Drew (Community Service)—

he interrupted me to tell a story about a UCLA medical student who professed throughout his time at UCLA his commitment to the underserved. Several years after his graduation, a member of the dean's team who was visiting alumni went to the office of this former student. His first surprise was that the office was in such an affluent community. Signs directed patients' paths: if you feel anxious, go to the right; if depressed, go to the left. Further down, signs said: if you earn more than $250,000, go left; if less, go right. The associate dean, of course, went right and found himself back outside on the street.

My parents had a way of inspiring us to high achievement in school. My mother made it very clear that even if she did not understand the math I was taking, she expected me to understand it, and to perform well. The ability to set expectations is a quality that I've valued as a leader, and as I've worked to help others develop as leaders.

As the Community Health Leadership Program at the Satcher Health Leadership Institute interacts with mayors and other community leaders, I am impressed with the courage and commitment that allow them to take on such difficult positions. As we try to support them in their health leadership roles, it is with great admiration for them as leaders in communities where they must deal with poverty, violence, and discrimination. They often take great career risks in assuming these roles.

Leaders must certainly be decisive, even when all the information is not available to them. Growing up on a small farm in Anniston, Alabama, where the availability of food and water was often dependent on the weather, our decisions to plant crops were often made with incomplete information. Over the years, I came to appreciate how well my parents negotiated these conditions. Certainly making decisions in times of uncertainty is a function of leadership, and it is a skill not easily taught. Developing trusting relationships and clear communication are key to working through such challenges.

When I think back over my career, especially when leading historically black colleges and universities with skimpy budgets, I appreciate the need for leaders to make decisions in the face of uncertainty. They say that necessity is the mother of invention—I can tell you that when leading an HBCU, the need for innovation is paramount. In making critical allocation decisions regarding budgets and expenditures, much has to be balanced. We cannot compromise on the quality of education students receive in their classroom or laboratory experience.

When I called Secretary of Health and Human Services Donna Shalala about the release of *Healthy People 2010*,[2] on a snowy morning in January 2000, she did not have time to get all the information before deciding if we should go forward, since the meeting would begin within three hours. But a decision had to be made, and we made it, releasing the Healthy People 2010 agenda as scheduled.

Of all the qualities of leadership, the one I find most encompassing and impactful is that *leaders must be able to respond to opportunities, challenges, and even crises.* In the final analysis, it is how leaders respond that will determine their place in history. Among other things, this means that leaders do not have an equal opportunity for success or failure, because they do not all respond to the same imperatives. They are dealing with varying opportunities, challenges, and crises. Lincoln had to respond to the Civil War,[3] Franklin D. Roosevelt to World War II,[4] and Reagan to the breakup of the Soviet Union.[5] Barack Obama had to respond to being the first black president and all that that implied,[6] and to a health system that was imperiled, with over 40 million uninsured people.[7]

Embodied within these challenges are opportunities to succeed impressively or fail miserably. It is one thing to look at a challenge from the perspective of the president of the United States, or even of a major college or university. But what about parents whose interventions may determine if their children survive, or if their brain development is properly stimulated by good nutrition and early communication?

Eighty percent of the parents in the Smart and Secure Children's Program at SHLI are single parents. Many of them have several children, with very little support. As leaders of their families, by joining the program, they already demonstrate one of the most important qualities of leadership: a willingness to learn more about parenting and more about themselves as parents.

Dr. Walter Fluker, who served as a member of the SHLI/MSM faculty in its early days, in his book *Ethical Leadership: The Quest for Character, Civility, and Community,*[8] defines *integrity* as trustworthiness and the ability to honestly face oneself, one's deficiencies, and one's obligations. Integrity means thinking about yourself and others individually. It involves leaders having a conversation with themselves in which they ask questions such as, Who am I? What do I stand for? Where do I stand? Can I be trusted to be who I say I am and do what I say I will do? Another question that leaders should ask themselves is, Am I committed to being the best that I can be, to being my best self physically, mentally, and yes, spiritually? Am I committed to healthy living and lifetime habits of physical activity, good nutrition, avoidance of toxins, sexual responsibility, and stress management? All these things are needed for leaders to be their best selves and to make the most of the resources they have been given. It is interesting that integrity includes a commitment to make the best of oneself. In short, we have been endowed physically, mentally, and spiritually with certain capabilities, and it is up to us to develop those to our highest potential.

Civility deals with how we treat other people—whether or not we treat other people with respect. The first question leaders should ask themselves is, Do I have a healthy respect for others regardless of their status on our team or their station in life? We owe other human beings a level of respect. And of course, we will generally find that if we treat other people with respect, we will get the same in return.

In many ways I think the term *civil rights* exemplifies this priority. The civil rights movement was about the quest for civility of treatment[9]—the right to get the best education, to socialize, and to work without regard to race, creed, or color. It was about having the right to achieve one's full potential without being discriminated against in the process.

Community is the third aspect of ethical leadership as discussed in Dr. Fluker's book. It starts with the spirit of community—that which brings us together around shared goals and values. It includes acting in the best interest of the community and working with the community to develop standards of behavior and service. It also includes seeing ourselves as having a responsibility for and within the community, and regardless of our status, seeing ourselves as part of the communities in which we live, work, and serve. One of the greatest failures of leadership is to think that it is "all about me" rather than the cause or the mission. The spirit of community allows us to build homes, schools, churches, and indeed businesses or even nations. The same spirit will allow us to build a health system that serves everyone with quality and dignity.

When partnerships are formed for the common good of everyone, we have community in the best sense of the word. That is the spirit of community, the realization that it takes working together to make a difference for families and individuals. Working together, a group can ensure quality education, safe environments, and livable wages for everybody. But none of these benefits of community action is likely unless someone leads the way.

I have often been asked what was so special about Dr. Martin Luther King Jr. and his ability to communicate. Many people, after hearing Dr. King speak, were not only informed but also ready to act. Dr. King had the ability to paint the picture for people, even if they had little formal education, and to do it in a way that was clear to them. It is important to point out that Dr. King had a doctorate from Boston University and that he often used what we call "big words." However, even when he used such words, people understood what he was talking about and what he needed from them. He had an amazing gift, and to a certain extent, leaders need to be able to educate, motivate, and mobilize, though not necessarily as well as Dr. King.

Leaders should trust their intuition but also, based on it, have a clear vision and plans for where it is trying to take them, how they will get there, and how they will know when they have arrived. The vision of the Morehouse School of Medicine, "Leading in the creation and advancement of health equity," is a clear statement of where the institution should be heading and where it would like to be in the distant future. A clear vision allows us to set appropriate goals and objectives.

Leaders must know themselves and continue to learn about themselves. The experience I had as a child, with whooping cough and pneumonia, and the suffering involved with that, including the struggle to breathe, created in me a level of self-awareness that has remained throughout my life and my career. I had to get in touch with myself during the struggle with this severe disease, and I have come to believe that most people who suffer severe illnesses, especially as children, have a level of self-awareness that serves them well in leadership roles. It is my experience that many physicians suffered certain illnesses as children. But for those who did not, it helps to work to understand those who did or do suffer such experiences. Many people have become more in touch with themselves when they have watched loved ones suffer from certain illnesses and become incapacitated or perhaps die. Others gain this sensitivity when they serve as volunteers in hospitals, nursing homes, or similar facilities.

Leaders must be able to overcome their own egos. Leaders who engage the team approach to leadership rely upon the expertise of other members of the team, for example, in areas such as budgeting and fund-raising.

Again, Dr. Benjamin Elijah Mays served as president of Morehouse College for twenty-seven years and interacted with many students as he spoke in chapel every Tuesday morning. Today, Morehouse graduates all over the world still quote Dr. Mays. He certainly was able to educate, motivate, and mobilize us to work toward the achievement of higher ground. As stated earlier, Dr. King, like his mentor Dr. Mays, had an unusual ability to communicate with people at all levels, all over the world. In Montgomery, Alabama, with the world as a stage, he was able to mobilize people to nonviolent action.

On the farm and in the foundry where I also worked, my dad often led by example—the way he responded to responsibility and the way he treated other people. His example still defines who I am and how I behave. A very important quality of leadership is that we behave so that others can learn by watching us and by what we do, not just what we say.

While I was president of Meharry Medical College, from 1982 until the end of 1993, the survival of the institution was always in question. The financial situation was threatening, especially because of the growing hospital debt, and the fact that our programs had been excluded from public funding.

Today's leaders face many challenges as members of a global

society. Those challenges require an understanding of diversity as never before. At the same time, they will provide an opportunity for new discoveries and for leaders to take advantage of expertise and knowledge that is held globally. With a broad perspective and effective leadership, we can move toward the vision of health equity.

Chapter Seven

Discipline in the Quest for Health Equity

To lead in the quest for health equity, individuals and members of groups must be disciplined. How we eat, sleep, drink, handle relationships with others, and how we manage power, all reflect our discipline. One of the first lessons I learned in my life was that I could not take life for granted. Whooping cough, contracted at an early age, taught me that I could not take breathing for granted, either. What I remember most about it was struggling to breathe. Because of that, my earliest memories in life relate to these struggles to breathe. When I finally recovered from whooping cough, I knew that I would not take breathing or life for granted ever again.

In time, it became clear to me that I had a responsibility to help others get free and stay free of disease. Long before I knew the phrase "disparities in health,"[1] I knew that health was not equally distributed.

I was surprised, during my eleventh year as president of Meharry Medical College, to receive a call to interview for the position of director of the Centers for Disease Control and Prevention. I had long admired the work of the CDC, especially their goal of helping children, worldwide, to achieve optimal health. But my career had not been in public health practice. My major interest represented a blending of public health and medicine, or community medicine. I had had the opportunity to work with a giant in that field, Dr. M. Alfred Haynes, with whom I served as a Macy Faculty Fellow at the King/Drew Medical Center and at UCLA. Our focus was on the Watts community[2]—one of the most challenging underserved communities in America. Watts had poverty, violence, and a distinct lack of access to health care. I went there to work for two years and ended up staying seven. I gained a reputation in community medicine, working especially with hypertension and sickle cell disease. I started a free clinic in the basement of a church, while running a primary care residency. The work gave me the opportunity to develop models of care and community health promotion and to share what we learned in national journals.

The morning of the interview for the CDC directorship I had volunteered to assist elementary school teachers by serving as a positive role model for their students in a project of the newly developed 100 Black Men of America organization,[3] which I had helped to start and develop. I felt no particular pressure about the interview, because it was not a position that I had ever envisioned myself holding.

On that particular morning, I had taken some kids into the hallway of the school to help them with reading. While in the hallway, I noticed tobacco smoke. I expressed concern and asked the kids about it. They told me that some of the teachers smoked in the break room. When I asked the teacher with whom I was working about it, she explained that the exhaust vent had not been working for several months. I could not believe it. These young kids were being exposed to tobacco smoke at a tender age, and while in school at that. Neither the message nor the experience could be tolerated. They were being shown that it was okay to smoke, and they were being exposed to the toxins in tobacco. I have always been slow to anger, but I was infuriated.

When I returned to my office, I had forgotten about the interview, which was about to take place. I didn't even know that some of the country's leading epidemiologists in the public health profession would be on that call. They included the assistant secretary for health, Dr. Phillip Lee; Dr. Bill Foege, who led in the eradication of smallpox; and Dr. Donald Hopkins, a fellow Morehouse graduate, who was leading an effort to eradicate guinea worm disease. When the interview started, I was out of control. I could only think about the kids at that school. When they asked me important public health questions, I would come back to those kids and their exposure to tobacco smoke from teachers smoking in the break room. I was convinced that there was something wrong with a public health system that could not protect children or persuade teachers to quit smoking or help them resist starting in the first place. How can we begin to teach children discipline if their role models cannot exhibit it?

When the interview was over, I was convinced that I had blown it. I shared this with my wife, Nola, who reminded me that I was probably trying to do too much if I could not plan for such an important interview; she was right. But the next day, I received a call from Dr. Lee, the chair of the search committee. He said to me, "David, that was one of the greatest interviews that I have ever been a part of. We want you to come to Washington to interview with Secretary of Health and Human Services Donna Shalala." I was amazed! Apparently the committee felt that I had the kind of passion about the health of children that was needed at the CDC, considering that only 55 percent of American children were being immunized by the age of two and that too many communities like Watts and Detroit had less than 30 percent immunization rates. So I agreed. I was beginning to feel that maybe this was my next move, even though I was enjoying my position at Meharry more than ever, since we were having major successes in fund-raising and faculty recruitment and were moving toward the merger of Meharry Hubbard and Nashville General Hospitals.

I had never met Secretary Shalala, but I knew that she had previously been president of the University of Wisconsin. I did not know what to expect. This time I prepared by thinking about the points I wanted to make in this very important interview. When I walked into her office, she looked up at me and said, "So you're David Satcher?" and I said, "Yes, I am." She then asked, "Do you really want to be director of the CDC?" Without hesitation this time, I said yes. "Well, if you want the job, you have it. I have heard from the search committee, and they were unequivocal about you, and I have full confidence in that committee. I look forward to working with you." Just like that, my wife and I started planning for the next phase of our lives.

Public Health is "the collective effort of a society to create the conditions in which people can be healthy."[4] But successful public health requires individual and community discipline. It is a call for all of us to take responsibility for making the best of our lives and our health, and our ability to foster an environment that supports both.

Leaders have a responsibility to model individual and community discipline, in physical activity, nutrition, avoidance of toxins, sexual behavior, and sleeping practices. At the CDC, in 1996, as we approached the fiftieth anniversary of the agency, we acknowledged our responsibility as the global leader in public health. If we wanted America and the world to exercise discipline in physical activity, good nutrition, and the avoidance of toxins, the CDC needed to model that kind of discipline. And so, at the beginning of 1996, when I had been director for two years, we asked ourselves and our employees to join us in setting a healthy example for the world.

At the beginning, only about a third of the employees at the CDC were physically active on a regular basis, and even fewer claimed to consume three to five servings of fruits and vegetables per day. We decided to focus on these two measurable behaviors. We set up a system of competition among our various centers, institutes, and divisions. We changed the food choices in the cafeteria and gave an extra thirty minutes for lunch to those who wanted to be physically active. At the end of the year, we had doubled to 70 percent those who engaged in regular physical activities and consumed three to five servings of fruits and vegetables per day.

Later in 1996, the CDC worked with Acting Surgeon General Audrey Manley to develop and release *Physical Activity and Health: A Report of the Surgeon General*,[5] since we felt that this was the major deficit in the health behavior of the American people. At the time, we knew that less than a third of the American people were physically active on a regular basis. We also knew that there had been a major decrease in the percentage of schools requiring physical activity for K–12: less than 29 percent. In fact, between 1990 and 1995, it had decreased from 50 percent to 30 percent. At the same time, childhood obesity was increasing. Schools felt they needed more time for math and reading, and thus they felt comfortable taking time and experience away from physical activity. The Surgeon General's Report on physical activity recommended that schools return to K–12 physical activity and that all Americans engage in a regular program of physical activity at least thirty minutes a day, five days a week.

This report would form the basis of what would become the Surgeon General's Prescription,[6] when I became surgeon general. In addition to the recommendations for physical activity, I would add four more. If followed, we knew that those behaviors could prevent over half of the chronic diseases that were costing Americans so much in health care, illness, and death. But following the Surgeon General's Prescription (a recommendation from a Surgeon General's Report presented in a keynote address to a pharmaceutical group, later made into a handout that looks like a prescription) would require individual and family discipline; in fact, it would require community discipline—especially in terms of facilities and safety. In addition to the regular physical activity recommendation, we prescribed good nutrition. We could not spell out all of the details for good nutrition on the prescription, so we settled for what we felt was the most important nutritional recommendation: to consume at least three to five servings of fruits and vegetables per day. In retrospect, we probably should have said, "Start the day with a healthy breakfast, and consume at least three to five servings of fruits and vegetables per day." Our experience is that when fruits and vegetables in the diet are increased, fats and sweets in the diet almost invariably decrease.

The third recommendation was to avoid toxins, with a special focus on tobacco use—still the leading cause of preventable deaths in the nation. But we also warned against the use of illicit drugs, especially mind-altering drugs, and the abuse of alcohol.

On the fiftieth anniversary of the Surgeon General's Report on smoking and health,[7] we celebrated the fact that since its release in 1964, the percentage of Americans who smoke on a regular basis had decreased from 43 percent to 18 percent. That figure continues to drop and is now close to 15 percent. In the process, we estimate that more than 10 million American lives have been saved. However, as deaths continue from past and present smoking, we know that some 20 million deaths due to smoking have occurred in that last fifty-year period.[8]

The fourth area covered by the Surgeon General's Prescription was sexual health, which was perhaps the most difficult area to capture on a small prescription. After much and continuing debate, we recommended "responsible sexual behavior, including abstinence, where appropriate." Of all the items on the prescription, there are more questions about this one than any other. People continued to ask, What do you mean by abstinence, where appropriate? I usually respond by pointing out that young people need to know that sexual relations should not begin with sex, but with genuine human relationships. It is my contention that anything that stimulates conversation about sex and sexual health is worthwhile; so we continue to set an example, pushing the discussion when many others would shy away. In retrospect, I would have preferred a more specific prescription.

During a presentation in 2017, when I got to that recommendation, someone in the audience broke out in spontaneous applause. Later that gentleman came up to me and said that he had made a promise, and even a bet, that if I talked about sexual health in the presentation he would applaud, since it is so rarely included in any public discussions. Yet sexually transmitted diseases, including HIV/AIDS, syphilis, gonorrhea, and chlamydia continue to be major health problems in our society. More than that, marriages continue to struggle, and even dissolve, because couples have so many unanswered questions about sex. They still have trouble discussing that aspect of their relationship. Sexual health includes healthy communications about sex, especially for married couples and couples who are committed to each other's well-being and pleasure. The language of item four on the prescription has been revised a few times, as we continue to improve communication about human sexuality and sexual health.

Self-discipline in the area of relationships between different genders is especially challenging for many. Inappropriate behaviors can destroy relationships, families, and even businesses and institutions. To help assure appropriate discipline, every supervisor needs an advisor; every mentor, in fact, needs a mentor.

Outside of committed relationships, appropriate communication between people of different genders is critical when power is not equal. It has certainly been said that power is a great aphrodisiac, and thus leaders must be responsible to control their own behavior, especially with people who report to them, even when these people invite attention. The responsibility for assuring that such relationships remain professional requires special discipline on the part of leaders.

Finally, the Surgeon General's Prescription speaks to a very important need for all of us to "calm down"—the need to relax physically, mentally, emotionally, and spiritually. One of the great challenges to our health and well-being is stress, and the need to manage stress is paramount. If we do not manage stress, then stress will manage us. When we allow stress to get the better of us, it is at a great cost to our total health and well-being.[9]

Stress is especially injurious to our nervous system. It saps our energy and interferes with sleep. Our prescription recommended seven to nine hours of sleep per day, which is critical for optimal functioning. Stress is an adversary with a strong sense of irony: it increases the need for sleep, while interfering with our ability to sleep.

We cannot leave the prevention or the management of stress to chance. We must be intentional about planning relaxation and managing the stress in our lives. It is worth repeating: If we do not manage stress, it will manage us. Stress interferes with our sexual health, and thus our sexual relations, creating more stress not only for individuals but for couples in relationships, as well. Mental health problems, such as anxiety and depression, also increase as stress increases.

Stress interferes with performance in general, including performance in the workplace. In short, in order to be most productive in our work, we must be disciplined in managing our stress. This requires the management of our schedules and our relationships. We must build relaxation into our schedules, and we must make sure that time with family and friends is on our schedules—unless of course, those relationships, as they sometimes are, are the source of stress. We should define and seek out stress-reducing or relaxing relationships and interactions. Perhaps ironically, we must be disciplined in our planned relaxations. If we are not careful, even our disciplined schedules will manage us. In most cases, the secret to a disciplined and yet relaxing life is balance.

For most of my life, I have been a long-distance runner; I ran distance in college. When I got to medical school, I struggled with a rigorous curriculum, in an environment where African Americans represented less than 2 percent of the student body: the pressure was on. So I gave up my disciplined running program to devote more time to study. That was a mistake. I would later learn that I studied more efficiently when I was on a running program. I got by in my academic performance, but it was in the second semester that I returned to my running program and excelled in medical school as I had in college.

Clearly, running for me has been a major strategy for relaxation and managing stress. But after training for and running the Marine Corps Marathon in my last year as surgeon general, I realized I had reached a point at which running could become more of a burden than a source of relaxation. Thus, I have become more disciplined in balancing running, walking, rowing, reading, listening to music, and watching movies. Some would add aging to that balance equation, although I certainly have less control over that component. Healthy aging is certainly enhanced by a balanced program of physical activity, nutrition, avoidance of toxins, and responsible sexual behavior.

In many ways, leadership discipline is more challenging than individual discipline. But of course all of us are, first and foremost, individuals. Leaders, however, are responsible for managing several very important relationships: first, the leadership team, then beyond the team to other internal institutional relationships; and second, relationships with external individuals and organizations, including vital partnerships. In order to be optimally disciplined as a leader, we must be well-informed about the opportunities and challenges facing us, both as individuals and as leaders of organizations.

Chapter Eight

Leading from Science to Policy to Practice

PRECEDING TODAY'S PROGRAMS is a long history of more than a hundred years of development, of testing and evaluating, and of constant research to provide the best in nutrition, nutrition education, and food service for the nation's millions of children in school."[1] This statement was made in 1971 by Gordon W. Gunderson, who worked with the United States Department of Agriculture to establish school lunch programs during World War II. It demonstrates the importance of science to policy making, and policy making to practice, and how the three interact, over time, to define and redefine goals and how best to achieve them.

Science, at its best, often leads to changes in policy at the community level, but policy change does not always lead to changes in practice. This is illustrated by the Gunderson quotation. For example, we were pleased when the Local School Wellness Policy was established by the Child Nutrition and WIC Reauthorization Act of 2004,[2,3] and later the Healthy Hunger-Free Kids Act of 2010.[4] These policies promised physical education in grades K–12 and healthy foods in schools, especially for students receiving free lunch and free breakfast. However, many schools still do not provide K–12 physical education or nutritious meals.[5] When challenged, their claim is that they lack resources, including funds to hire physical education teachers. The School Health Policies and Programs Study 2006 revealed that between 2000 and 2006,[6] the percentage of school districts that had adopted a policy stating that schools will follow national, state, or district physical activity standards had risen from 66.5 percent to 81.4 percent.

But science alone cannot shape policies. Policy is also influenced by politics, opinions, deeply held beliefs, and advocacy. As surgeon general, I based all fourteen of my reports on the best available public health science.[7] Yet, the Surgeon General's Report does not always lead to a change in policy; sometimes it takes years for that to happen. For example, after the release of *Smoking and Health* in 1964,[8] it was not until 1972 that tobacco advertising was prohibited.[9] Then, in 1995, California became the first state to prohibit smoking in public places, and as of March 8, 2019, twenty-eight states have such laws.[10] In some cases, cities within states have different policies, despite the clear signs of dangers from second-hand smoke.[11]

In the case of immunizations, where federal policy now covers access for children, regardless of their ability to pay, some parents deny the science of the policy and refuse to have their children immunized.[12] They have deeply held beliefs about the dangers of immunizations, in spite of reports, from the highest level of neuroscientists, that immunization involves no risk. Patients must be listened to and given the information that will enable them to make decisions based on real science, not on conjecture.

Sometimes it is important to continue to mount the scientific data and arguments in order to achieve policy change. As director of the Centers for Disease Control and Prevention, I was impressed with the work of some of our outstanding scientists. For example, Dr. Godfrey Oakley, an award-winning epidemiologist, pediatrician, and geneticist, conducted the study that clearly showed that augmenting folic acid in the diet of pregnant women reduced the incidence of neural tube defects in children,[13] but it took years to get policy consistent with that science. In 1995, I spent two weeks with Godfrey in China, examining data collected by our colleagues in Beijing, where neural tube defects were much more common than in the United States. The China Study,[14] a collaboration between the CDC and the Peking University Health Science Center, showed that augmenting the diet of pregnant women with folic acid had clearly reduced the incidence of neural tube defects—by almost 90 percent in some areas of China. Yet it was not until 1999 that the US Congress passed legislation supporting the fortification of flour and meal with folic acid,[15] leading to the beginning of a dramatic reduction in neural tube defects, such as spina bifida, in the United States.

In 2009, the Commission on Social Determinants of Health of the World Health Organization (CSDH/WHO)[16]—a commission on which I served—reported, after a worldwide study, that social determinants of health (SDH) had a much greater impact on health outcomes than did health care. We defined SDH as the conditions into which people are born, live, grow, learn, work, age, and die. These conditions are controlled by money, power, and influence and can only be changed when policies that impact them are changed. For example, many low-income, predominantly black neighborhoods often lack grocery stores and markets that sell affordable fruits and vegetables and other nutritious foods. Predominantly white neighborhoods have four times as many supermarkets as predominantly black neighborhoods.[17] We know that people who live in these communities are more likely to suffer from obesity and diabetes and other diet-related problems than people who live in communities where healthy and nutritious food is readily available.[18]

The state of Pennsylvania addressed its concern about areas where citizens lacked access to fruits and vegetables by creating, in 2003, the first economic development initiative in the country "aimed at improving access to healthy food in underserved rural and urban communities."[19] Known as the Fresh Food Financing Initiative, it supports the development of new stores in underserved urban and rural communities across Pennsylvania. In addition to providing underserved communities with new stores, the initiative also created a significant number of jobs for local residents.

The Affordable Care Act included the work of the National Prevention, Health Promotion. and Public Health Council, which proposed a National Prevention Strategy,[20,21] based primarily on the objectives of *Healthy People 2020*.[22] It would assure all children access to safe places to play, in order to develop lifetime habits of physical activity. However, Congress has consistently refused to fund these provisions and has generally not supported the prevention agenda.

There are several points at which leadership can seek to intervene to improve the health of individuals and communities. These points are referred to as downstream, midstream, and upstream and are based on the McKinlay Model.[23] *Downstream* refers to individuals and the attempt to improve their health through education, science, and medicine. This is critical for dealing with practice as well as with science.

Midstream is at the level of community and community environments, seeking (1) to remove environmental threats to health— for example, lead and other toxins—that can severely impact child health and development; (2) to assure safe places for children and others to be physically active; and (3) to assure that community institutions, such as schools and workplaces, promote the health of those who use them. These community organizations and businesses can also provide incentives for workers to quit smoking or to engage in regular physical activity. By incentivizing its 100,000 employees to participate in wellness programs, Johnson & Johnson saved $225 per person per year in health care bills over a four-year period.[24]

Upstream is where policy is made that impacts what happens midstream and downstream. I try to emphasize that these are not places, but functions. Policies are often made in the home or school, not just in the houses of government. But the Surgeon General's Report should impact all of these settings based on the best available science.

When I released the Surgeon General's Prescription in 2000,[25] it was an attempt to inform Americans and urge them to be more physically active, to consume more fruits and vegetables, less fats and sweets, and to avoid toxins such as tobacco and illicit drugs. However, it is clear to me now that the best way to deal with these behaviors is to remove barriers and to provide incentives for physical activity, good nutrition, and smoking cessation, as well as to assure that communities are safe and that they provide the facilities that individuals need to live healthy lives.

Clearly, communities can restrain or enhance healthy behaviors and can prohibit smoking in public places. This led to that dramatic decrease in smoking in California, mentioned earlier. In 2001, when I released the Surgeon General's Report on women and smoking,[26] California was the only state in the union in which lung cancer deaths were not increasing among women,[27] perhaps due to the state's aggressive campaign against smoking in public places. But the arrow goes both ways: from upstream to downstream, and from downstream to upstream. What happens downstream, whether science, practice, health care, or education, can lead to enhancements in policies from upstream. Thus, leaders must intervene appropriately at every level and ultimately assure that the right policies are in place and that they are consistent with practice.

The Quality Parenting Program at the Satcher Health Leadership Institute at the Morehouse School of Medicine is evaluated for its impact on the parent and child participants.[28] We hope the findings will influence policy and lead to investments that will improve the plight of children, their development, and their readiness for school. Thus, a practice downstream, when properly evaluated, can improve policies upstream. The NIH has already responded to outcome data showing a reduction in depression among the black female parents in the program, and has supported the replication of this quality program in twelve states, primarily in the southeastern United States. Hopefully, we are on the path to proving that investment in enhancing quality parenting is a great policy position, one that makes a difference in our communities.

Public health and public health science are especially important to improving the health of communities. The CDC foundation defines *public health* as "the science of protecting and improving the health of families and communities through promotion of healthy lifestyles, research for disease and injury prevention and detection and control of infectious diseases."[29] In 1988, the Institute of Medicine's report, *The Future of Public Health*, defined *public health* as "the collective efforts of a society to create the conditions in which people can be healthy."[30] Whereas *public health* is also often defined as "the state of health of the public or group of people," I prefer the IOM definition, understanding that "the conditions" rely on the right policies being in place. Even with the newfound appreciation for the importance of social determinants of health, the definition of public health takes on new significance, as does the public health approach that involves the following four steps:[31] (1) define the problem, (2) identify risk and protective factors, (3) develop and test prevention strategies, and (4) assure widespread adoption.

As mentioned in Chapter 2, in 2005, colleagues and I published an article entitled *"What If We Were Equal?"* in the *Journal of Health Affairs*,[32] in which we attempted to define the problem of disparities in health in the United States by looking at data comparing African Americans with whites in terms of mortality rates. These are the two groups for which we have the most data, going back for a century. We were able to show that if mortality rates had been equal for African Americans and whites in the twentieth century, then in the year 2000 alone, there would have been 83,500 fewer deaths among African Americans. We were able to clearly define the magnitude of disparities in health in terms of mortality outcomes. We then examined the major determinants of health in four major categories: genetics, health care quality and access, environment (physical and social), and behavior.

In a 1993 article in *JAMA*,[33] McGinnis and Foege showed the relative impact of these four areas of determinants, with behavior accounting for over 40 percent of the variation in outcomes, compared to 25 percent for environment, 20 percent for genetics, and 10 to 15 percent for health care. However, given the WHO Commission on Social Determinants of Health Report, we are forced to revisit the issues of determinants of health and to look more carefully at the conditions that impact these four areas. Relative physical inactivity is virtually predetermined in communities that are not safe or lack safe places to be physically active, just as the absence of grocery stores limits access to fresh fruits and vegetables.

The major difference between the goals of *Healthy People 2010* and *Healthy People 2020* is that *Healthy People 2020* incorporates the SDH in terms of problems and solutions.[34,35] In this sense, the definition of public health from the 1980s preempted the report of the CSDH by focusing on "the collective efforts of a society to create the conditions by which people can be healthy." Armed with this new perspective, the WHO felt that it was time to set the goal of "global health equity" and to begin to work toward that goal. This is important, and in keeping with it, the SHLI/MSM has as its vision "to become a transformative force for global health equity."

In 2002, the Ford Foundation funded the Morehouse School of Medicine National Center for Primary Care to lead a National Advisory Council consensus panel on the topic of sexual health and well-being,[36] as a follow-up to the Surgeon General's Report on sexual health in 2001.[37] We put together a balanced group of people, in terms of opinions and perspectives. About one-third of the participants were conservative relative to human sexuality, including Focus on the Family,[38] a global Christian ministry, and various church groups. Another third would be considered liberal and included SIECUS (Sexuality Information and Education Council of the United States).[39] The final third was moderate, and included members of the American Academy of Pediatrics, which is dedicated to the health of all children.[40]

At the outset, it was difficult to get everyone to agree to meet, since they had a history of antagonism. Some even brought bodyguards to the first meeting. Opinions were deep and strong, and relationships had to evolve. Some individuals ultimately became friends, even though they continued to disagree on some key issues. Three areas of agreement were reached after eighteen months. First, the group agreed on a vision for sexual health in America; second, on the importance of parents as sexuality educators for their children; and third, on the need for more funding for research into human sexuality and sexual health. The group published a Consensus Report,[41] and recently, two members of my staff, Sharon Rachel and Christian Thrasher, along with Dr. Robert Hatcher, professor emeritus of Emory University School of Medicine, published a book on sexuality education based on the group consensus on parents as important sexuality educators.[42]

Still there were key issues on which the group could not agree. They held firm to strong opinions in spite of science. This was especially true when it came to homosexuality. Science is clearly on the side of those who hold that homosexuality is not a choice, a selected lifestyle, but that individuals are born with the tendency toward homosexuality or transgender preferences.[43] For some people, however, homosexuality is contrary to deeply held religious beliefs. It was interesting that one of the most religiously conservative members of the group became good friends with the openly gay person who sat next to her in most meetings. There's something about human relations that sometimes defies explanation.

One must conclude that while science is critical to decision making, relative to the world around us, it is not definitive and thus does not have the final word in debates dealing with sexuality or even climate change. There is still the need for people to come together, listen to and hear each other, and try to arrive at reasonable decisions that promote societal health.

It is, however, critical that we continue to do the science, and to repeat studies, because science at its best is repeatable, even when carried out by different people, at different times, in different places, as long as conditions can be standardized. But scientists are not considered to have a lock on truths. When people come together to make important decisions or to invest significant resources, they generally want to know what the science shows. Thus science requires persistence, patience, and determination.

From Science—It is because of science that we have vaccines that have eliminated diseases from populations and even eradicated a major disease, smallpox.[44] It is because of science that we have reduced deaths from both cardiovascular disease and cancer and diabetes.[45,46] It is because of science that we are able to help people with "unquiet" minds, such as bipolar disease, to lead productive lives when given the right medications.

The Science—Science is certainly important in policy making. The Surgeons General's Reports are based on the best available public health science—not politics, not religion, not personal opinion. So the release of the Surgeon General's Report *Smoking and Health* in 1964 led to a series of policies meant to protect the American people from smoking and to shield them from exposure to smoking and smoking-related behaviors that could lead to addiction. But a Surgeon General's Report is not meant to be the final word; it is the latest word. Science must continue. Even though the first report on smoking and health had an impact, it was not until 1972, when *The Health Consequences of Smoking: A Report of the Surgeon General* was released,[47] that the danger of secondhand smoke was recognized. It was even later that science determined that almost 90 percent of adult smokers became addicted by age 18,[48] a finding that led to a policy forbidding the sale of tobacco to children.[49]

Although the Surgeon General's Report of 1964 showed that smoking was associated with lung cancer and heart disease, we have continued to learn more about the harmful effects of smoking. In 2014, when the fiftieth anniversary Surgeon General's Report was released,[50] at least six new health defects associated with smoking were reported.

To Policy—Likewise, as we have learned more from scientific research related to smoking, new policies have been established or made. In the 1970s, President Richard Nixon signed a law banning the advertisement of tobacco on television and radio.[51]

To Practice—In 1995, California became the first state to outlaw smoking in public places. By 2000, when I released the Surgeon General's Report on women and smoking, California was the only state where lung cancer was not increasing in women.

This dynamic interaction among science, policy, and practice is basic to progress in lifestyle and healthy living. In the area of smoking and health, we have perhaps had the most experience and made the most progress. Even though science never ends, there comes a point at which the evidence is strong enough to declare that our practices need to better adapt to our current science. After years of research suggesting the dangers of smoking, and especially its role in increasing the risk for lung cancer and cardiovascular disease, Surgeon General Luther L. Terry declared in 1964 that there was overwhelming evidence of a causative connection between smoking and lung cancer and cardiovascular disease. This declaration led to new policies and new practices, such that smoking in the United States had declined from 42 percent in 1965 to 14 percent in 2017.[52] We estimated that between ten and twenty million lives had been saved due to smoking cessation or the decrease in smoking initiation. As we write this, the decline continues, not only in our country, but globally.

In 2003, it was the World Health Organization Framework Convention on Tobacco Control,[53] a global tobacco control treaty, that led to a global policy related to exposure of children to smoking. One hundred eighty countries found the six science-based strategies, known as MPOWER, adequately tested and accepted them. MPOWER is an acronym for Monitoring tobacco use and prevention policies, Protecting people from tobacco smoke, Offering help to quit tobacco use, Warning about the dangers of tobacco, Enforcing bans on tobacco advertising, promotion, and sponsorship, and Raising taxes on tobacco.[54] Now, even in developing countries, smoking is declining and lives are being saved because of a decrease in smoking in public places. Today the decline in smoking is a global phenomenon, because science builds on science over the years and over the ages. Nevertheless, I am certain that there are still people who don't agree that smoking is harmful to health.

Policies are not, however, made on the basis of science alone.

They are also influenced by deeply held beliefs, by money, and certainly by the political process. The practice of smoking has not been easy to influence, despite the science. Yet, the CDC's Office of Smoking and Health assembles the science, and each new Surgeon General's Report imparts this new information on the basis of the latest scientific developments. As we observe practice in society, we keep looking for messages from science that keep us moving toward more smoking cessation and less initiation of smoking. This is, appropriately, a circular process of new science, new policy, better practices, and new questions arising from observation and practice.

It is in the operation of science—science, policy, and practice—that the leadership role of the surgeon general is defined. However, no report from the surgeon general can be issued without a clear basis in science. Scientists from the CDC, the NIH, Substance Abuse and Mental Health Services Administration (SAMHSA), and others must develop and act on the science in order for an official report from the surgeon general to be issued. But the question that gives rise to the science may begin with a practice as the basis of concern, or it may be a policy that is in question, and those concerns and questions often lead to new science.

The dramatic decline in physical education in the schools between 1980 and 2000 was thought to be good for academic rigor and performance. Upon closer examination, however, a dramatic increase in obesity was taking place, including a tripling among children. The science also revealed that children who were physically active and ate a good breakfast performed better academically! Thus, examination of practice and the policies behind them revealed that they were out of step with good science. The Surgeon General's Report not only revealed a connection between sedentary lifestyles and obesity but also showed that the former was not consistent with good academic performance. *Physical Activity and Health: A Report of the Surgeon General*, in 1996, and *The Surgeon General's Call to*

Action to Prevent and Decrease Overweight and Obesity, in 2001,[55] documented this and called for an increase in physical activities and a decrease in sugary caloric intake.

In the 2001 Surgeon General's Report on childhood obesity, changes were recommended based on the accompanying care, or communication process, research, and evaluation. The settings for this intervention were to be homes, schools, communities, workplaces, and health care settings. In order to make an impact, the Surgeon General's Reports must reach and interact with all of these settings and continue to modify the science, the policies, and the practices. In the face of the best available science, it is often difficult to get the right policies in place—that's the job for the surgeon general. As we have seen with obesity and smoking, we often need the surgeon general and his or her reports to intervene. Likewise, when practices are not consistent with science or policies, the surgeon general is often most influential. Trust is also a major factor in his or her effectiveness, and when it is not there, the job is significantly compromised.

While pursuing my MD and PhD degrees, I came to appreciate both the differences and similarities between the two programs. I've often said that in preparing for the practice of medicine, we had to learn the guidelines for successful practice, or to recognize the lines, and walk them, but in preparing for the research career, we had to learn to draw the lines, and walk them too. Like most assertions, this is not entirely true, but it's a fair assessment of important distinctions between preparing for medical research and preparing to practice medicine, both of which I have enjoyed. Science is rigorous and begins by defining critical questions for pursuit. We are allowed to propose our hypotheses, but we can accept them only after we have rigorously tested them. Science never ends: one set of questions generally leads to testing and the proposition of another set of questions.

Medicine is a science in the sense that we are committed to practice it in a way that is consistent with the state of science; we never stop asking questions, and over time our practice improves. Today we do not diagnose or treat diabetes and hypertension the way we did when I was a student. We have developed new science, and it has reshaped our practice. However, between science and practice, we develop and attempt to follow policy guidelines. Using these guidelines, the Food and Drug Administration regulates the practice of medicine.

One of the beauties of science is that it is always open to questions, debates, and challenges. The scientific process must always be open, and it must always be opening new horizons in our minds, in our lives, and in our environments.

Chapter Nine

Confronting the Epidemic of Overweight and Obesity

A s we approached the end of the twentieth century, it was obvious that overweight and obesity were growing at epidemic proportions, especially in our children.[1] While the term *epidemic* has generally been reserved for infectious disease outbreaks, such as polio, lime disease, measles, and Ebola, we felt it was appropriately applied to what was happening relative to childhood obesity. Use of this term for the increase in obesity was first applied by public health leaders at the CDC.[2] When the prevalence or incidence of a disease is increasing rapidly, far beyond what would be expected, we call this an epidemic. It may be influenza, HIV/AIDS, whooping cough, or measles. When an epidemic occurs, we attempt to respond with appropriate alarm, intervening forces, immunization regulations, and at times quarantine—all in an effort to curtail the continued spread of the problem.

In the mid to late 1990s, we noticed that childhood overweight and obesity had doubled since 1980. We also knew that a child who was overweight or obese at age 12 had a great risk (80%) of being overweight or obese as an adult, and was also at risk for the associated problems of diabetes, heart disease, hypertension, and others. In an attempt to spark action, we released *The Surgeon General's Call to Action to Prevent and Decrease Overweight and Obesity* in 2001.[3] Importantly, in the report we used the word *epidemic*.

While the report included specific guidelines for confronting this epidemic, it was clearly not going to be a short-term intervention, and it was essential that we begin a vigorous response. Unlike other Surgeon's General Reports, we also issued guidelines that were targeted to different settings that engaged children in activity and good nutrition. These settings included the home, community, school, health care, and workplace, all of which had a major role to play in containing the epidemic of overweight and obesity.

It was not enough, we felt, to feel good about what we were doing; we needed to measure the impact of our actions on the epidemic. This is especially important in dealing with children of different backgrounds, whether it be culture, race, social economic status, or educational level. We could not afford to lump children of different races and ethnic groups together in such a way that we missed specific strengths, challenges, or needs. By measuring disparities and the magnitude of the problem, disparities in participation, and disparities in outcomes, we are able to target interventions to the specific needs of these groups.

Although my tenure in government came to an end in February 2002, the year after the report on overweight and obesity had been released, in many ways my work in dealing with issues that I cared about did not end, but took on a new beginning. There were people and organizations that cared deeply and had resources to invest in combating these problems. It seemed there was always someone willing to invest in leadership by providing resources for the struggle.

Even before I left government, the National Dairy Council sought my help in identifying programs they could invest in to confront overweight and obesity in children. Not long after I left government, the National Dairy Council held a national conference in Washington, DC, to discuss the problem. Parents, community leaders, health planners, teachers, and other school officials were invited to that meeting, and most invitees came. Earlier, as president of Meharry Medical College, I had experience in organizing national conferences—one of which led to the creation of the *Journal of Health Care for the Poor and Underserved*.[4]

Out of that first meeting, a national program called Action for Healthy Kids,[5] or AFHK, was developed. It was headquartered in Chicago, home of our first CEO, but had spread rapidly throughout the state and, to some extent, the nation. It has had quality leadership at both the board and the staff levels. But, despite significant financial support, its funding was not keeping up with the demands for its programs, so it sought a better fund-raising strategy. I agreed to serve as board chair, and we recruited outstanding staffing. While we were concerned about the experience of children in all of the five settings identified (family, community, school, workplace, and health care), we were able to gain the most traction in schools, where children spend more supervised time than anywhere else. Schools were also a major contributor to the problem of childhood obesity; most had reduced physical activity or physical education and served high caloric foods in the cafeteria.

It was pointed out in *Physical Activity and Health: A Report of the Surgeon General*,[6] released in 1996, that between 1990 and 1995 the proportion of schools requiring K–12 physical education dropped from 50 percent to 30 percent. It was a dramatic change. Schools worried that programs in physical education were taking time and resources away from teaching reading and math, on which they were critically evaluated. One of the most important reports issued by Action for Healthy Kids was the 2005 annual report, which provided evidence that children who were physically active and consumed a healthy breakfast did better in school—results in reading, math, and standardized exams were all better—and were better disciplined. Together, the National Dairy Council and the National Football League contributed over $200 million for enhancing physical education and good nutrition in 14,000 schools and for 38 million students.

Even though Congress passed the Local School Wellness Policy in 2004,[7] urging schools to return to physical education K–12 and to target good nutrition, the money was still not made available in most school districts in the country. Although this was an actual policy, it did not become a universal practice. Because of increased attention on the issue, however, and growing numbers of integrative strategies, physical education was integrated into math and other classes, and obstacle courses that required meaningful physical activity confronted some children as they got off school buses in the mornings. But there is still a major deficiency in physical activity in schools' curricula.

Drawing attention to the issue also led Congress to pass the Healthy Hunger-Free Kids Act in 2010,[8] specifying the type of foods to be included in the school lunch and free meal programs. Innovative strategies, such as Grab and Go, which packages healthy meals in small packages, made it easy for kids to get a healthy breakfast and ameliorated the shame some kids feel about receiving free meals, since these packages were available to all who wanted them.

In 2008, the National Dairy Council and the National Football League decided to develop a foundation to support programs such as Action for Healthy Kids and on-site school programs. I credit this to interaction among certain board members. When you attract one outstanding person to a board, he or she attracts others. The National Dairy Council helped to involve the secretary of Agriculture, and that led to others. The release of the Surgeon General's Report stimulated great interest and involvement. While I was in the process of stepping down as board chair, I was asked to join the board of this newly created GENYOUth Foundation,[9] which included the chair of the NDC and the commissioner of the NFL, among others. Since 2008, almost a billion dollars have been raised for the activities of the GENYOUth Foundation. Most of the funding has come from the National Football League Foundation and the National Dairy Council. The signature program is the Fuel Up to Play 60 program,[10] which pushes children toward eating a healthy breakfast and being physically active for at least sixty minutes a day. More than 38,000 schools are participating in the program, and some 14 million children are now being supported by it. I am most impressed by the emphasis of Fuel Up to Play 60 on student leadership. In 2016, during Super Bowl week, we rewarded student programs that were most innovative and had the greatest impact. At the end of 2016, I announced my resignation from the board of GENYOUth Foundation, but I continue to be excited about what is happening throughout the country and will be available when needed to support these efforts.

Because I had called out the problems of childhood overweight and obesity as surgeon general, other leadership demands and opportunities continued to present themselves to me in these areas. In 2012, then new governor Nathan Deal started the Georgia SHAPE initiative as Georgia's response to the epidemic of child overweight and obesity.[11] He asked me to serve on the SHAPE board. Since Georgia is my home, and I was serving on the faculty of the Morehouse School of Medicine, I felt it was not only a leadership opportunity but a responsibility. Agreeing to serve on a board or boards represents a commitment to work to improve one's community. We all have a responsibility to respond to these kinds of requests, but it also helps to spread our influence. Georgia ranked in the top 5 percent of states in terms of childhood obesity and overweight. We obviously had a major problem. On the board, I would work with the then Georgia commissioner of the Department of Public Health, Dr. Brenda Fitzgerald, a board-certified obstetrician and gynecologist and a fellow in anti-aging medicine. She had practiced medicine for over three decades before becoming commissioner and was named director of the CDC in 2017, replacing Dr. Tom Frieden. Other leaders on the board included Co-Chair John Bare of the Arthur Blank Foundation, which had a major interest in childhood behavior, as well as other educators and pediatricians. Governor Deal's SHAPE program is a network of partners, agencies, the Georgia Department of Education, and even athletic teams, including the Atlanta Falcons and the Atlanta Braves, all committed to improving the health of Georgia's children by offering assistance and opportunities for them to achieve a high level of overall fitness.

I like SHAPE's focus on fitness in students, beginning with a basic benchmark called the FITNESSGRAM, to monitor fitness annually. The assessment includes the evaluation of five components of health-related fitness—aerobic capacity, muscular strength, endurance, flexibility, and body composition—all using objective criteria. Reports are generated that provide valuable individual, school, and state-level data. The reports are made available confidentially to families, and aggregated results are reported to create a "true" snapshot and to highlight areas of improvement. Having this information empowers parents, schools, and communities to assess the current health needs of their children. I particularly like that the program is not just targeting children with problems of overweight and obesity, but rather the behaviors that relate to these problems. This program engages all children to compete against themselves, in terms of fitness goals. It is fair to say that we are beginning to see progress, and that the increase in overweight and obesity seen in the last two decades of the twentieth century has been curtailed. Nationally, Georgia is no longer in the top 5 percent, but now ranks nineteenth, with a pattern of progress we plan to continue.

I was recently asked to be lead author of an article in *Public Health Reports* outlining Georgia's strategy and progress. I was pleased to do so because publishing is an important part of leadership, as we try to share with our colleagues ideas that can "lift all boats."

In the National Center for Primary Care at the Morehouse School of Medicine, and then later at the leadership institute, we ran a program called Community Voices: Healthcare for the Underserved,[12] which targets, among other things, the problem of overweight and obesity in both children and adults. Through the program we took on the challenges involved in enhancing community support, including health care, healthy lifestyles, as well as access to health care and supportive, healthy environments. Achievement of these goals often requires influencing and changing policies. Some municipalities have developed new policies and programs that support and promote locating venues with fresh fruits and vegetables within the reach of all its citizens.

The leadership institute also houses a Health Leadership Development Program, which brings community leaders and health leaders together to develop team strategies for improving the health of the communities they serve. This program has been in existence for over seven years, and has included pastors, church members, nurses' aides, City Council members, and county commissioners. Ten mayors have graduated from this program. My view has always been that mayors are on the front line of the major challenges of violence, poverty, and overweight and obesity, which often go together. For example, it is unrealistic to expect people to engage in physical activities if their communities are unsafe for walking or jogging, and there are no parks available for children to play in. Our communities must be supportive of healthy behaviors. Every child should have access to healthy food and access to safe places to be physically active.

With the help of one of our first mayoral students, Mayor Johnny Ford, former mayor of Tuskegee, Alabama, and with the help of the Marguerite Casey Foundation, we developed a community health leadership program specifically for mayors. We know there is value when mayors get together with other leaders, and we are going to make sure that continues to be the case. We appreciate the opportunity the Marguerite Casey Foundation has given us to better target mayors and to develop strategies for making these programs work. I have found that successful fund-raising usually results from combining a good strategy with a good reputation for prior successes.

Often, corporations are in an ideal position to provide incentives for healthy behavioral change. For example, Johnson & Johnson, which has over 100,000 employees, provides health insurance for most of its employees and their families. In a 2010 *Harvard Business Review* article, the CEO of Johnson & Johnson documented the mutual beneficial impact of smoking cessation and weight loss among its employees.[13] Since this company is self-insured, its cost is lower when its employees are healthier and engaged in healthy behavior. Amazingly, by helping their employees quit smoking and lose weight, Johnson & Johnson realized cost savings of well over $100 million a year. There's also growing evidence that healthier lifestyles among the employees rubbed off on their families and community. This workplace program provided an excellent opportunity to impact the health of the company by improving the health of the employees and their families, thereby decreasing the cost of medical care.

It is tempting to take for granted the role of physicians and other health care providers in working to curtail the epidemic of overweight and obesity. Given all the documented connections between overweight and obesity in childhood and obesity in adulthood, it is clear that a wakeup call is needed for the health care system to intervene as early as possible. We know from our work with smoking and health that health care professionals do not always make prevention and health promotion a major part of their agenda. Thus, it is crucial that we take every opportunity to urge health professionals to not only discuss the importance of good nutrition and regular physical activity with their patients and their families but also, when appropriate, to actually write prescriptions for exercise and healthy eating. The Surgeon General's Prescription was intended to be a model for others to use.

Medical societies, such as the American Society of Pediatrics and the Academy of Family Medicine, must increasingly incorporate behavioral change as a part of their programs of continuing education. I am very pleased to see that, as with the Surgeon General's Prescription,[14] which calls for physical activity at least thirty minutes a day, five days a week, many providers are now actually writing prescriptions for behavioral change. In each of these roles, it's important to find ways to lead toward health equity. I do not take for granted the opportunities I have had to lead, but with each of these opportunities has come responsibilities that most people do not necessarily have.

Needless to say, the struggle against the epidemic of overweight and obesity is a long-distance race, and, like the battle against infectious disease, it will require long-term vigilance. Since there is not a vaccine for overweight and obesity, we will need to change the way we behave, including the way we eat, what we eat, our physical habits, and other behaviors. It will require cooperation and coordination among home, community, schools, and workplace, together with the health care system. However, it is perhaps most important that medical education itself include directions for helping patients to engage in healthy lifestyles. The failure to include the importance of healthy lifestyles in medical education is a failure to instill the value of health promotion and disease prevention. Otherwise, the attitudes of future physicians are being shaped for a health care system that is ultimately unaffordable and increasingly inhumane.

At every level in the struggle for health equity, if we are to be successful, we must have leaders who can communicate, coordinate, evaluate, and motivate. Somehow, we must speak and act with one voice about the importance of physical activity and good nutrition. The earlier these messages and interactions are implemented, the more likely we will be to prevent the continued increase in over-weight and obesity and such associated problems as diabetes, heart disease, hypertension, and cancer.

Culture will also be important in this effort. Our goal is not to stigmatize people who are overweight and obese, because everyone is not at equal risk. Our goal must be to help everyone achieve his or her best weight and to minimize obesity. The FITNESSGRAM approach used by the Georgia SHAPE initiative is a healthy approach because it challenges everyone to work toward and achieve optimal fitness, which is different for different people. Cultural differences also impact the appropriate nature of our intervention. While excess salt in a diet must not be acceptable in any group, we must work to find the appropriate taste for people of different cultures. "Soul food" must not be an excuse for consuming excess salt, since we know the impact of such diets on blood pressure, especially in African Americans, who have a higher risk of developing high blood pressure than any other ethnic group.[15]

It is the responsibility of health care providers to understand the culture of each patient and how it impacts his or her health behaviors. With that understanding, doctors can lead their patients to a healthier lifestyle, including food, dance, and general movement. The Integrated Care Model,[16] which has been developed for mental health, and is showing significant progress as an intervention, is relevant for weight control. To the extent that we are able to integrate the community into our programs to control and achieve healthy weight, our efforts will be realistic and effective. We need people on the health care team who understand the resources of any community, and who understand how people can and will move in order to fight obesity and achieve optimal weight. The greater our knowledge of what brings people together in a community, the more we can integrate healthy behaviors into these gatherings.

I am reminded of one of the early fellows in the SHLI Health Policy Leadership Development Program. When she moved into a new community, she sought to continue her habit of early morning walking or jogging. However, she was warned by members of the community that it was not safe for a young lady to walk or jog in the early morning. She became a leader and called the community to-gether to find out if others were interested in early morning physi-cal activity. She brought a group together and organized a walking group; in numbers, they found safety. Local law enforcement offi-cers even took notice and made plans to patrol the area in the early mornings. Thus, one person became a leader and changed an en-tire community in terms of safety and healthy behaviors.

Perhaps no issue has been a greater challenge and opportunity than the problem of overweight and obesity. First, scientists at the CDC defined the problem as an epidemic, even though no chronic disease had been defined as an epidemic before. Next, it was up to leaders to heed the advice of the experts. This is why I've said that listening is the most important form of communication for leaders.

Because surgeons general listen intently to the science of an issue, their reports are not based on personal opinions or beliefs, but on the best available science, which they trust as a basis for new policies and practice. That trust, which starts with listening, is in-valuable. The sciences are never final, but always open to new ob-servations, new evidence, new explanations, and new theories. As we work to implement new programs, we must continue to evaluate the impact of interventions and be open to new findings, new explanations, and new data.

Listening alone is not enough; leaders must also respond. Leaders must respond most assiduously to the science, but also to the concerns of the community and of the leadership team. There will be both opportunities and challenges to any response, no matter how clear the right path may seem. Leaders must respond to opportunities to mobilize groups of people in communities. By continuing the response at every level, this type of leadership can improve the health of communities for years to come.

Perhaps in no area are the social determinants of health more important than with the problem of overweight and obesity. We have defined the SDH as "the conditions in which people are born, grow, learn, work, and age."[17] We also know that social determinants of health are influenced by the distribution of resources in society. To the extent that one has the resources to live in communities that are safe, communities that have ready access to parks and other places for children and adults to engage in healthy behaviors, then one is more likely to be healthy.

We have said that in order to make changes in the SDH, we will need to make changes in policies. Certainly, one of the most important responsibilities of leadership, including that of the surgeon general, is to try to change policies that are not contributing to the health of the community. But that's not the end of the effort. We need to follow through to ensure that policies lead to the appropriate changes in practice. Obesity is a perfect example. We have identified an epidemic and instituted programs to combat it. Together we must continue to learn the nature and magnitude of the problem and the opportunities we have to achieve a society of optimal weight, based on optimal nutrition and behavior. We can thus prevent a lot of pain and suffering.

Chapter Ten

The Advancement of Reproductive Health

T HE MISSION OF PUBLIC HEALTH, "the collective efforts of a society to create the conditions in which people can be healthy,"[1] can be seen clearly in reproductive health. In
fact, it takes more than a collective; it takes a strong community to
deal with issues in reproductive health. Perhaps no area of health
policy has been more controversial and more challenging than this
one. It is appropriate that we have available well-developed public
health teams, working to assure the health of women, of mothers,
and of babies. It is certainly one of the most important investments
that can be made locally and globally. And yet, at the same time, it
is a topic of much debate, in which the impact of culture can be
almost overwhelming.

Reproductive health involves the health of women from menarche through menopause,[2] the health of women and others during
pregnancy, as well as the health of the newborn infant. Even though

not all women have children, a great deal of their physical, mental, and social interactions relate to preparing for and responding to reproductive experiences. Thus, all of the forces that impact the health of women during this period of time must be considered a part of reproductive health.

The social determinants of health (SDH), including education, income, health, poverty, violence, even religion, and certainly access to health care, are all critical to reproductive health outcomes. These factors are reflected in infant mortality and maternal mortality and morbidity. Perhaps in no area of public health do we see the impact of social determinants of health more clearly than in reproductive health. We could go on; the conditions in which pregnancies take place also often include unsafe water, infectious diseases, and most important, lack of educational opportunities for girls before, during, and after pregnancy.

Pregnancy and its outcomes are often a focal point. As the various changes associated with pregnancy take place in a woman's body, they challenge her basic health. When pregnancies are not planned, the risk of things going wrong is increased. Teenage pregnancy (15–19 years) carries a slightly higher risk for mortality and other problems than pregnancies among 20- to 24-year-olds.[3] Women older than 35 have the highest maternal mortality rates. Teenage pregnancies are usually not planned and often not wanted. Teenagers also tend to be less knowledgeable about their bodies and the need for health care, nutrition, and physical activity. Teen pregnancies are often associated with poverty and low levels of education, and culture and socioeconomic status also play an essential role.

Maternal mortality globally accounts for close to 300,000 deaths per year,[4] and even in high-income countries like the United States, we continue to be challenged. We've made only slight progress in reproductive health since the turn of the century. It is appropriate that when we want to compare different countries in terms of health and health care systems, we tend to prioritize infant mortality or the rate of death of children in the first year of life. This is certainly a most delicate period, and it reflects so many ways in which babies' health can be damaged. Among these are genetic risk factors for diseases, including cystic fibrosis and sickle cell disease. I worked with sickle cell disease during the early part of my career, and among other things, coauthored a book dealing with counseling and the importance of parents being aware of how the disease is transmitted. Sickle cell genetic counseling certainly does not advise parents whether or not to have a baby based on the risk, but it seeks to ensure that parents are prepared to deal with the outcome of pregnancies. It makes a difference for the health of the baby and the health of the family. But all the forces of public health ultimately conspire to get a baby through the first year of life, and many of these collective activities must take place before the baby is born. Access to good nutrition, clean water, prenatal care (including contraception), and genetic testing are critical for giving babies the best chance in life.

The fact that the United States ranks below many developing countries in infant mortality is a concern for us all,[5] especially those of us in public health. That places such as Cuba and Bermuda have better health outcomes for infants than we do should be a major concern for our country.[6] It's not that we haven't made progress. In fact, from 1965 to 2015, there was a reduction in infant mortality of around 74 percent—but we're not keeping up,[7] and we have the opportunity to do so much better.

Other developed countries and even some much less developed than we are do better than we do when it comes to keeping babies healthy. That should not be acceptable. It should also concern us that there is great disparity within our nation when it comes to infant mortality. If we raised our worst outcomes to our own average outcomes, we would certainly rank much higher among the nations of the world. Without taking anything away from anybody, we have the opportunity to create equity of access and quality, and to do it in such a way that we raise the bar for everybody. As we recognized at the fiftieth anniversary of the Division of Reproductive Health at the CDC in 2017, we have much to celebrate.[8]

In 1996, I agreed to join the YMCA on a trip to Southeastern Africa to participate in a project geared toward making clean, safe water more available, especially to women and children. In addition, we were concerned about the growing spread of HIV/AIDS and wanted to get a better understanding of what could be done to help slow the epidemic. We had planned visits to Zambia, Tanzania, Zimbabwe, and Kenya. I took the opportunity for a side trip to Malawi, whose president was Dr. Hastings K. Banda—a graduate of Meharry Medical College. Dr. Banda was a very popular alumnus, and on one occasion he was responsible for the largest gift ever received from an alumnus. Faculty, alumni, and students alike were very proud of Dr. Banda. I was eager to meet him for many reasons, not just his generosity to Meharry, although that certainly was a factor.

Malawi, a country of macadamia nut trees and beautiful lakes, was exhilarating. I especially enjoyed getting out and walking in the morning among the trees and along the lake. Dr. Banda was interested in my visiting his major source of pride, the Queen Elizabeth Hospital, which he had built. For Africa, it had relatively modern facilities and technology, including a 250-bed Ob/Gyn unit.

It was an impressive structure, and it sparkled with cleanliness and order. There were no data regarding outcomes, but it was striking that 90 percent of the patients on the Ob/Gyn unit were teenagers who were delivering or were in the immediate postpartum period. I asked the medical director and others about the problem of teenage pregnancy, and how they were dealing with it. Clearly, they had difficulty understanding what I meant by teenage pregnancy as a problem. At that time in their culture, women were generally not allowed to attend school beyond the sixth grade, and it was expected that teenagers would marry early, sometimes into families where husbands had more than one wife. Because of their culture, my question did not go over well.

The Malawi experience worried me because in many cases, neither the teenage body nor the teenage mind is adequately prepared for pregnancy. The maternal mortality rate is generally higher in Africa than in other countries, and it seemed clear that teen pregnancy was a factor. For example, in 2008 the maternal mortality rate was 1140.1 per 100,000 live births in Malawi compared to 16.6 per 100,000 in the United States.[9] It was a stark and dismaying difference. So we had an opportunity to intervene, to improve the health of women, and thus improve the health of pregnancies, babies, and families. I reflected on our work back in Nashville, where Meharry Medical College, under the leadership of the head of Ob/ Gyn, Dr. Henry Foster, would later win one of President Bush's Points of Light awards for the school's work to prevent teenage pregnancy and increase the high school graduation rate.[10]

Later, after returning to Zambia, I visited the United Nations International Children's Emergency Fund (UNICEF)[11]—one of my favorite global organizations. When I told them about my trip to Malawi, and especially to Queen Elizabeth's Hospital, they related the relevance of my experience to one of their major concerns— the rapid spread of HIV/AIDS. They said that in their opinion, the best or most important thing that could happen to reduce the spread of HIV/AIDS in Africa would be the education of women, so they would not only know how to protect themselves, but they would also have greater control and independence relative to men in their society. For example, one man with HIV/AIDS will often spread the disease to ten or more women.

Certainly, over the last twenty years, we have seen these educational opportunities for women expand in Africa, and even HIV prevention programs such as loveLife,[12] in South Africa, funded by the Kaiser Family Foundation, seem to be making a tremendous difference, not only in AIDS control, but in women's health generally. Years later, when I was serving as surgeon general, one of my assignments was to work with the South African minister of health, as part of the agreement between Vice President Al Gore and South African Deputy President Thabo Mbeki.[13] I was pleased to find that, even though it has the highest rate of new HIV cases in the world, South Africa had already come a long way.[14]

Even in the United States we have a long way to go to reach optimal sexual health education. Recently, I participated in two ceremonies where endowed chairs were established in the name of former Surgeon General Joycelyn Elders, one at the University of Minnesota, where she did her residency training, and another at the University of Arkansas. In 1994, after serving less than two years as the surgeon general, Dr. Elders was forced by President Clinton to resign from her position for her bold and outspoken approach to sexual health education.[15] A reporter had asked her whether masturbation should be taught in schools, and Dr. Elders responded that it should certainly be considered. People should know how to manage their sexuality, she thought, and it was already known that she had suggested a far greater distribution of condoms in high schools.

Dr. Elders has always spoken openly about having been fired, and she has never held a grudge or negative attitude about her firing or about President Clinton. She understood that President Clinton fired her rather than run the political risk of her outspokenness. And yet, it is gratifying that more than fifteen years later, Dr. Elders is being honored for her courage, her outspokenness, and her clarity.

Clearly, Dr. Elders and her plight reflect the general problem with sexual health and reproductive health in the United States. In many ways, we are hypocritical about our behavior and in what we're willing to share with our children, teenagers especially, about sexuality. Knowledge that might save them from premature pregnancy or even death from a disease like HIV/AIDS is considered impolitic, even among public health's allies.

When I became surgeon general in 1998, I was mindful that Surgeon General Elders had been fired because of her public discussion of sex, including masturbation and the use of condoms. But, I was determined that there needed to be a well-thought-out Surgeon General's Report on sexual health based on the best available science. Although I was appointed by the Clinton administration and served my first three years with President Clinton, *The Surgeon General's Call to Action to Promote Sexual Health and Responsible Sexual Behavior* was finally released during my last year,[16] when I served under President Bush. I must say that it was not easy to get the report released because as a nation, we still have difficulty openly discussing issues related to sex and sexuality. The secretary of Health and Human Services did not attend the release of the report, and I understood why—but he allowed it to happen.

While President Bush never expressed support for a Surgeon General's Report on sexual health, he clearly also allowed it to happen. Secretary of Health and Human Services Tommy Thompson said, "The American people need to read that report."[17] However, as the time drew near for me to release the report, I spent an uncomfortable two hours responding to questions from members of Secretary Thompson's staff, including scientists with expertise in reproductive health. They wanted to know if the report would stand the test of time and the test of science. They read it carefully and asked me tough questions. I was joined in that meeting by my deputy surgeon general, Dr. Ken Moritsugu; we acquitted ourselves well and were allowed to release the report. I will always appreciate Secretary Thompson and President Bush for allowing us to release the report on their watch. It is also interesting that President

George W. Bush (to my surprise) would later support the President's Emergency Plan for AIDS Relief.[18] He is now quite proud of this program, which has done so much to slow the spread of AIDS in Africa and to improve treatment.

Here in the United States, however, we still have difficulty dealing with the topic of sexual health, so most of our schools are not allowed to discuss human sexuality, even though teenage pregnancy, sexually transmitted infections, and sexual violence remain major problems. Clearly, deeply held beliefs are sometimes more powerful than science when it comes to sexual health and sexual education policy.

After I left government, the Ford Foundation supported a consensus-building program in which twenty-four people from various organizations—equal numbers of liberals, moderates, and conservatives—were brought together. The Consensus Report,[19] which was developed later, revealed three areas where this very diverse group was able to find common ground. One was to develop a vision for sexual health that included physical, mental, and sexual health. The program provided a valuable experience and issued an important and valuable report. Since that time, another important book, *Sexual Etiquette 101 & More*,[20] has been written by two of my former assistants at the Morehouse School of Medicine and Emory Professor Emeritus Dr. Robert Hatcher.

We have been told that our willingness to develop and release a report on sexual health after a previous surgeon general had been fired for discussing the topic represented strong leadership. I released several reports from the Office of the Surgeon General, four of which are relevant to reproductive health, even though not obviously about that topic. In addition to *Tobacco Use among U.S. Racial/Ethnic Minority Groups*,[21] and *Reducing Tobacco Use*,[22] the report *Women and Smoking* was released in 2001.[23] Among other things, we now know that smoking increases the risks associated with pregnancy and can damage the reproductive organs, as well as many (if not all) other organs. Even the report on oral health included information about the impact of periodontal disease on the reproductive health system.[24] Of course, the Surgeon General's Report on overweight and obesity[25] continues to be important because chronic diseases, such as hypertension and other heart-related diseases, increase with overweight and obesity, and they can impact pregnancy and delivery and increase risks during this time in a woman's life.

Whereas we have made major progress in smoking and health, and saved an estimated 10 million lives since the Surgeon General's Report of 1964 on smoking and health,[26,27] we still have miles to go in the areas of overweight and obesity. We have to continue to provide the kind of leadership that will allow us to overcome this problem. Likewise, the progress that has been made in the prevention of end-stage renal disease in the Native American population is promising in relationship to reproductive health. Progress in diagnosis and treatment of HIV/AIDS is also progress in reproductive health, and so we must continue to lead in all of these areas.

The three Surgeon General's Reports on mental health, including the landmark first-ever report on mental health,[28] treating children with mental illness,[29] and *Mental Health: Culture, Race, and Ethnicity* all have implications for pregnancy and reproductive health.[30] For example, depression in and around pregnancy and the postpartum period is a problem that we continue to struggle with, but hopefully, as we become more aggressive at diagnosing and treating mental health problems, we will be able to reduce their severity and magnitude.

Whether it is diabetes, hypertension, HIV/AIDS, or many other diseases, the impact and the implications for reproductive health can be significant. Protecting and advancing the health of women in many dimensions has a major bearing on reproductive health. Where there are disparities in the health of women during this time of life, there are disparities in reproductive health experiences and outcomes. As long as there are disparities in wealth, there will be disparities in health, especially reproductive health. As long as there are disparities in the social determinants of health generally, there will be disparities in health. Disparities in education, wealth, income, safety, and access to health care will continue to lead to disparities in health, including safe and full-term pregnancies, and disparities in maternal and infant mortality.

The importance of a healthy start in life is too often not appreciated. In some segments of our population, we allow for preterm deliveries to become the norm, and healthy outcomes are often dependent on heroic efforts on the part of the health care team. My colleague Dr. Henry Foster cited as one of his major disappointments that we have not been able to do a better job of bringing babies to full term and avoiding many of the health challenges that result from early deliveries.

During my time at the CDC, several things happened that I am proud to reminisce about. Some of them relate to women's health, some to improving pregnancy outcomes, and certainly some to the health of babies; significant progress has been made. I'm proud that we were able to appoint the first female deputy director of the CDC, Claire Broome, at a time when there had not been a woman in that kind of leadership role at the CDC, even at the level of its institutes and centers. An outstanding scientist, Dr. Broome had been involved, as an Epidemic Intelligence Service officer in the late 1970s and early '80s in discovering toxic shock syndrome, a problem caused by *Staphylococcus aureus* and the inappropriate use of tampons.[31] Her work moved us forward significantly in keeping young women healthy during this time of their lives.

When I appointed Claire as deputy director, she was eight months pregnant. Among other things, she led the development of a breast milk–pumping center, so that new mothers could breast-feed their infants uninterruptedly. She also led our response to one of the most difficult issues at the agency—multiple and disparate HIV/AIDS programs. She appointed a committee that recommended bringing all our HIV/AIDS programs into the National Center for HIV/STD and TB. An outstanding leader in so many ways, Dr. Broome was certainly more relevant to women in the childbearing years than any man could be. She was one of our best scientists, and I was very fortunate to have her as deputy director, especially as I had come from outside the CDC. I brought a new perspective to the CDC but clearly needed help from someone who had spent much of her career there.

We also had the opportunity to bring eight disparate HIV/AIDS programs together in the National Center for HIV/AIDS, Viral Hepatitis, STD, and TB Prevention.[32] This recommendation came from a group of people Claire and I had appointed to look at these programs to see where there might be a potential for better coordination. Helene Gayle was appointed to head the new center, where she served for six years, and she went on to do many great things in public health at the Gates Foundation,[33] as head of Global AIDS, and later as head of CARE.[34] More recently, she served as head of the Social Issues Programs at McKinsey.[35] Drs. Broome, Gayle, and Oakley are all examples of the opportunity to foster leadership among those who work under you and the importance of supporting it.

The passion of CDC scientists often led the way. Such was the case with Godfrey Oakley and his lifetime commitment to preventing tube defects in babies.[36] Neural tube defects include spina bifida and anencephaly. I traveled with Dr. Oakley to China in 1995 to learn more about the impact of fortifying foods with folic acid as a way of reducing neural tube defects—defects that were much more common in China than in the United States. As a result of our work, we were able to get the FDA to approve fortification of meal and flour in this country with legislation passed in 1999,[36] and since then we have seen a dramatic decline in neural tube defects. One of Godfrey's colleagues in China was an 84-year-old pediatrician who had spent much of her life and career working with this problem. The cooperation among scientists in China and the United States really demonstrated the potential for working together in a program to improve the health and the lives of people, especially babies. It was impressive.

It was, however, the appointment of outstanding women to leadership roles at the CDC that represented the greatest move forward for the institution and for my leadership there. I will always be grateful to those who supported this effort. Since that time, the CDC (under President George W. Bush) appointed a woman, Julie Gerberding,[37] to direct the agency.

Perhaps the most important thing that a leader can do to advance policy and practice is to appoint a strong leadership team, and I will always be proud of the team I had as director of the CDC. Each was an expert in his or her area, and I felt adequately informed and prepared, even when dealing with a challenging Congress. Even though I was the first black director of the CDC, I did not want that to be the issue. Instead, I targeted the role of women.

I thought it appropriate that the World Health Organization Commission on Social Determinants of Health,[38] a twenty-four-person commission, with representatives from diverse countries, on which I served for more than four years, begin its work by visiting Santiago, Chile. It was during the visit to Chile, in February 2005, our first official visit as commissioners, that we were formally introduced by the WHO Director General Dr. J. W. Lee.

Chile had developed a program that targeted SDH to improve access to education, especially for girls and women, since teenage pregnancy was a major barrier to the completion of high school for many girls. Chile decided to remove that barrier by providing daycare from the age of three months through the mothers' ninth grade.

The first three months of life are optimal for mother/child bonding, and care during that period should be encouraged. After the ninth grade, the need for daycare decreases considerably.

This program became a model that I think has resulted in a lot of progress, especially for women in Chile. Even in the face of teenage pregnancy, girls were expected to stay in school and finish their education. Not only did this program dramatically reduce school dropouts, it also reduced teen pregnancy. It enhanced the role of women in Chile, seeing them move rapidly into leadership roles, including the presidency. By targeting teen pregnancy and its impact on education, the entire society benefited.

This reminded me again of my experience in Africa, especially Malawi in 1986, where education for girls and women beyond the sixth grade was not encouraged, and teenage pregnancy was not seen as a problem but almost expected. It is important to point out that there was a difference in culture, and that it is unwise to judge others based on one's own culture.

There ought to be some standards of human rights that are universal—the right of girls to be educated and to make the best of their lives should be beyond reproach. In my opinion, the most important social determinants of health are education, income, and safety from violence. There are others, but these have always stood out for me. Just as there are global rules about the use of nuclear weapons, there ought to be such rules to protect children and prevent discrimination based on gender. When the AIDS epidemic spreads in Africa, it rapidly becomes a global concern, as does Ebola. Three million children dying of unclean water per year globally is a similar concern.

In cities such as Washington, DC, and Chicago, there are wide gaps (17–20 years) in life expectancy from one part of town to the next. These gaps relate to income and education of the population. Violence is too often most common among the poor.

Generally, I believe we are making progress. But we have not yet reached the level of confidence and integrity, when it comes to human sexuality and sexual health, that is needed for us to educate our children and to keep our children safe from themselves and from others, and to appropriately deal with the threats of HIV/AIDS and other sexually related infectious diseases. In order to continue to make progress in reproductive health, we need better science; we need better policies; and we need better practices at every level. We must attack disparities in health at every level and assure access to quality care for women from menarche to menopause.

When there are major differences in perspectives based on differences in worldview or deeply held beliefs or policies, we must find a way to work to bring hope for best practices to the table, even when some compromise is needed to bring that about. But we should also pause and meditate on the ways in which we can make our health system more responsive to the needs of all the people in the United States. By eliminating disparities in health in the wealthiest country in the world, we can certainly change the status of our health system for the better. We must be committed to that, and at the same time, committed to global health equity.

Chapter Eleven

Overcoming the Stigma of Mental Health Problems

G ETTING FROM SCIENCE to policy and practice can be greatly hampered by stigma. When negative attitudes and shame prevent individuals or their families from acknowledging an illness, those affected often fail to seek early diagnosis and treatment. That's one way stigma becomes a major barrier to prevention, early diagnosis, and treatment of disease. This is especially true of mental disorders. In the Surgeon General's Report *Mental Health*,[1] we reported that stigma impacted our dealing with mental illness in at least three or four ways. First, stigma prevented individuals from acknowledging their mental health problems and thus prevented early diagnosis and treatment. Likewise, family members, including parents, often neglect to seek care for a child with a mental disorder, due to embarrassment and even fear that such a diagnosis might interfere with the child's access to educational opportunities, as well as job opportunities later on.

In my own family, I can reflect on the struggle with mental illness that was not acknowledged. My cousin, who was about ten years older than me, had a tendency to run away from home. Once she was pregnant when she returned. The next time, she was dead when she was found. I often wonder if she could have been helped by care from a mental health specialist. But there were and are many barriers to care besides stigma.

Most disturbing, health care providers often fail to adequately assess the presence of mental disorders when carrying out what is supposed to be a thorough checkup.[2] But as Patrick Kennedy says in his book *A Common Struggle*,[3] "This often does not include a check-up from the neck-up, including the brain, the most important organ in the body." He describes a struggle that his and so many other families have with mental disorders. This is a book that could help to change the course of our work with mental disorders, I believe, by dramatically reducing the stigma often associated with mental illness.

Policy makers have allowed the health care system to discriminate in the assessment and care of mental illness. Often, people with mental disorders end up in the criminal justice system,[4] suffering punishment, rather than in the health care system, getting the care they need. In short, we dump our mental health problems into the criminal justice system. In recent years, some judges have taken the lead in assuring that people who come before them with behaviors betraying a mental health problem are sentenced to treatment of their mental illness and not just punishment for their aberrant behavior. These judges are making a tremendous contribution to health equity as well as to equal justice.

In November 1999, I had the opportunity to release the first ever Surgeon General's Report on mental health. The major recommendation was for parity of access to mental health services. It would take nine years of hard work with the Congress for the Mental Health Parity and Addiction Equity Act of 2008 to pass in 2008.[5] At Grady Hospital in Atlanta, patients with mental health emergencies waited as long as twelve hours to be seen. During that time they were often restrained. The introduction of integrated team care meant shortened waiting times and better care. It is interesting that leadership for the legislation, in both the House and the Senate, was bipartisan, and in each case was led by individuals who had experience with mental disorders in their own families. In the Senate, a very conservative Republican from New Mexico, Pete Domenici, sponsored the legislation, along with a very liberal Democrat from Minnesota, Paul Wellstone. What these senators had in common, again, was that each had a family member with a mental disorder and had had that experience growing up or watching their children grow up. Senator Wellstone would unfortunately die in a plane crash before the legislation was passed.[6] A strong advocate for the Parity Act, he was running for president when he died, with access to mental health parity as his major platform.

In the House, major support came from Patrick Kennedy, son of Senator Ted Kennedy and nephew of President John F. Kennedy. He fought tirelessly for passage of the legislation, and he is responsible for including addiction disorders in the bill. The Kennedy family has a long history with mental illness, and President Kennedy signed legislation in 1963 for the establishment of community mental health centers.[7] Even Patrick Kennedy himself has struggled with mental illness, especially with addiction. I began working with him while the mental health report was still being developed, and I have found him to be a great friend and ally in the battle for mental health parity and addiction equity. He is a gifted leader who cares deeply about this and other issues. In addition to caring, Patrick Kennedy is also quite knowledgeable and has the courage to act, persevering until the job is done.

In many ways I agree with Kennedy when he calls mental health "the civil rights issue of our times"[8]—especially in terms of the numbers of people affected, the discrimination, and the struggle. It is certainly true that people with mental illnesses are discriminated against today, as people of color were earlier and sometimes are today. Actress Glenn Close is also actively engaged in efforts to reduce stigma associated with mental health.[9] This has special significance for me, because it was during the student sit-in movement that I was arrested,[10] along with Dr. Martin Luther King Jr. and several students. While we were in jail, Coretta Scott King, Dr. King's wife, appealed to John F. Kennedy's campaign, fearing for her husband's life when he was abruptly and by night moved from the Atlanta jail to Albany, Georgia, where he had been arrested earlier. It was after a call from the Kennedy Campaign that Dr. King and the rest of us were released.

After the release of the report on mental health in 1999, I received letters and calls from people throughout the country, but one stood out. A young man in his early twenties wrote about his experience with stigma surrounding mental illness. His mother had died when he was eight years old, and her death was never discussed in his family. He finally figured out that she had committed suicide, but no one would discuss it with him. He thanked me for my report and wanted me to know that he was going to invite his family members to his home soon, and finally they were going to discuss his mother's suicide and the issue of mental illness in his family.

The struggle to get policy in place to assure access to mental health services continues, however, even after passage of the Mental Health Parity and Addiction Equity Act in 2008. In response to the law's requirement that mental health coverage offerings be equal to other coverage, many insurance companies decided not to cover mental health services at all, so as to bypass the parity requirements. It wasn't until the Affordable Care Act was passed in 2010 that mental health became an "essential health service."[11] This meant that mental health services had to be included as an essential health service by all insurance companies in all plans. This is a major step forward, especially for those covered by Medicaid, where discrimination in care is most common. Unfortunately, all states are not required to expand Medicaid.

Making mental health an essential health service represents a long overdue coming together of science and policy, but the struggle is not yet over. There's still a gap between policy and practice; many insurance companies discriminate in the actual coverage and reimbursement of mental health services, based on their own judgment of the appropriateness of services provided—which is in itself inappropriate. But, as with the civil rights movement,[12] things change when the law is on your side. Our greatest challenge now is to monitor the enforcement and practice of the Mental Health Parity and Addiction Equity Act, as they are not enforced throughout the country.

Each year, Patrick Kennedy and I conduct what we call a State of the Union in Mental Health and Addiction.[13] This event, which focuses on mental health parity and addiction equity, attracts people from throughout the nation. It provides an opportunity to assess what progress has been made in the reach for mental health parity and addiction equity, especially as it relates to the practice nationwide. It's a kind of monitoring that is required to assure that practice is consistent with science and policy. In many cases, it is not, and ongoing interventions are required. This issue is the major focus of the Kennedy Satcher Mental Health Policy and Research Center at the Satcher Health Leadership Institute.

Our attitude toward mental health is consistent with our attitudes and behavior toward the brain. Just as we often ignore the brain in the overall assessment of our health, and just as we often ignore its function, we ignore mental health. In many ways, the brain is the most neglected part of the body. For example, in many sports the brain is at risk, but the danger isn't acknowledged. It is not at all unusual for head-to-head contact to be the major focus of many sports. Boxing, football, soccer, hockey, and even basketball come with risks for the brain. Basketball can be especially risky for young women. Only in recent years have we begun to notice the aftermath of these sports' rough treatment of the brain. Former professional athletes are increasingly exhibiting signs of chronic traumatic encephalopathy, including memory loss, depression, anger, sleep disturbances.[14] Efforts are now under way in professional football and some other sports to better protect the brain. Leadership is beginning to come from coaches, parents, and even some fans— but not enough yet.

Some of us believe that our focus must be on prevention, which should start in childhood. With that in mind, the National Council on Youth Sports Safety was established a few years ago.[15] We know that over 300,000 children are diagnosed with concussions in emergency rooms each year,[16] and that the actual figure is probably much higher. We are convinced that the problem begins in childhood and that it is promoted by attitudes that ignore the safety needs of the brain. It is promoted by cultures, athletes themselves, parents, and communities that value competition, toughness, and winning more than safety. At a minimum, the brain is *ignored* in competitive environments. At worst, the brain is indirectly targeted. Clearly, this is an example of where our knowledge of the brain is being ignored.

Our goal was to develop a national alliance of youth sports safety, made up of athletes, coaches, trainers, parents, and community, where there is the commitment to develop a culture of prevention, one that will put the health of the brain above any other aspect of the game. Everyone who is now contributing to the problem must contribute to the solution if we are to be successful. That goal has not been achieved.

To the extent that the play of the game is inconsistent with pre-

venting concussions and related injuries, we must alter or amelio-
rate the game. Already, there is a National Federation of State High
School Associations coaches developing guidelines, describing what
every coach should know about concussions, and what every coach
should commit to do in response.[17] The board of this association is
headed by Jack Crowe, former coach at the University of Arkansas.
As we go forward with the alliance, we will have more and more
coaches committed to playing the games in a way that is consistent
with protecting the brain.

In our efforts to move from the best available science to policy
and practice, culture can play a prominent role, because in many
ways stigma is culturally based.[18] African Americans are only one-
half as likely to seek outpatient mental health services as the majority population. Asian Americans are only one-half as likely as African Americans to seek outpatient mental health services. American
Indians are twice as likely to be admitted to the inpatient services
as Caucasians, and they are almost never seen as outpatients.[19] Suicide in the American Indian population is generally much higher
than in the rest of the US population, and many suicides occur long
before mental disorders are diagnosed.[20] We believe that we can
change this by providing needed services in the community and
better engaging culture in our care system by involving an integrated team in promoting and providing the care.

About five years ago, after discussing this issue with the state of
Georgia, our leadership institute (SHLI) volunteered to take responsibility for mental health emergencies at Grady Memorial Hospital
in Atlanta—the largest public hospital in Georgia.[21] When we began
the project, a large percentage of patients would wait in the emergency room up to twelve hours to be seen by a psychiatrist on call,
and many patients had to be restrained while waiting. We developed an integrated team approach to care, engaging primary care
providers, social workers, physician assistants, nurses, nurse prac-

titioners, and mental health specialists, in a commitment to quality mental health care. Ongoing training is a major component to our commitment. As with our parenting program, training begins with the anatomy and functions of the brain and how these functions are enhanced by good nutrition and physical activity—including enhanced circulation in the brain after twenty minutes of exercise.

After two years, we had reduced waiting times by close to 80 percent and the use of restraints (both chemical and physical) by over 70 percent. Many of the patients were successfully engaged in a comprehensive continuity of care program, reducing visits to the emergency room. After three years, overall cost of mental health emergencies in Grady's emergency rooms had decreased by more than 40 percent. Providing better care at lower cost is possible when we remove the barriers to quality integrated care.[22] Similar models of integrated care also reduce the stigma of seeking and receiving mental health care, and there is also growing evidence that it improves the quality of care provided.[23] Integrated care greatly reduces the need for patients to be referred from the primary care clinic to another location for care. Then there is no need to call attention to the patient again. To make it work, training must be incorporated in the program on an ongoing basis. It is through training that the group can increasingly function as a team, all in the interest of improving the care of the patient.

The National Center for Primary Care at the Morehouse School of Medicine developed an acronym to place emphasis on the importance of culture as a component of quality care. It is called a CRASH course in cultural competence:[24]

- Consider culture
- Respect culture
- Assess culture
- Sensitivity to cultural differences

- Humility (recognizing that we will never be experts in other people's culture, and that we will at best be a student of that culture).

This acronym has served well to remind participants of the importance of culture in health care settings. In *Mental Health: Culture, Race, and Ethnicity: A Supplement to Mental Health: A Report of the Surgeon General*,[25] we pointed out that in health care settings, culture impacts both patients and providers. It impacts patients' willingness to seek care, often delaying care until it is quite late, and in the worst cases resulting in suicide before diagnosis. Culture also impacts the kind of care patients will seek. The level of stigma surrounding mental disorders varies from culture to culture.

Culture also impacts the provider and the nature of care provided, including diagnoses and treatment. A story from the Institute of Medicine report, *Unequal Treatment: Confronting Racial and Ethnic Disparities in Health Care*, describes how religion can influence how a patient responds to and communicates symptoms of mental illness.[26] Some religions see mental illness as being caused by "evil spirits" and not as a brain disease. According to the story, a black man who finally decided to seek treatment for an ongoing sad and gloomy disposition was referred to a prominent psychiatrist. When asked to describe how he felt, he stated that he often drove a truck cross-country, back and forth, and often felt as if the devil himself was sitting on the front seat with him. The psychiatrist interpreted the patient's description of his feelings to mean he was "seeing things" that were not there. Later, in the discussion, it became clear that the patient was quite religious and was describing his feelings in the context of his religion. The "devil" was his description of a very low and hopeless feeling.

The value of integrated care teams is that members who are not specialists may be in a better position to understand both the language and the cultural components of the communication. One approach to improving access to as well as quality of mental health services is to integrate mental health services into the culture of the patient. An integrated mental health care team may consist of one or more community health workers, a health educator, a nurse, a social worker, and a mental health specialist.

Each begins by learning about mental health and mental illness within the context of his or her own educational and expressed level, including how to respond to mental health emergencies. They are then integrated into teams with specific assignments based on levels of expertise.

After members understand their level of function and expertise and practice it, they are asked to respond to mental health problems as a team communicating with one another more and more, not unlike a sports team that begins by learning to play each position and then interacting with one another. This is, in part, the logic of the development of integrated teams at community health centers. Our Transdisciplinary Collaborative Center at the leadership institute studies the impact of community-based integrated care teams on access to and quality of mental health services.[27] Early indications are that, as at Grady Hospital, this strategy reduces the stigma that health professionals bring to health care settings and makes patients and families more comfortable seeking care. Cultural interaction reduces stigma.

As a medical student at Case Western Reserve University, I remember the first day of our Behavioral Health Services rotation (the name for our mental health experience). We were introduced to several patients on the ward. The patient who stood out was a 17-year-old black male, whom we discussed in the hallway, but we did not enter his room. He banged on the door, and we were told that he was violent. His diagnosis was paranoid schizophrenia. He was dark-skinned, and race was a major component of his paranoia. He did not trust white people, and he was violent. We were told that he would most likely be transferred to the state hospital, where he could be better managed. Out of curiosity, I asked if I could go back and visit with him later. The nurses warned that he was violent and that I should not go into his room, but the faculty gave me permission to do so, as long as I was "very careful." But he was a unique patient, and I gathered that the faculty wanted to learn more about him and to teach about a rare case of paranoid schizophrenia centered on race. The nurses offered to help, but would not take responsibility for my safety.

The next day, I went back to see the patient alone, with the nurses closing and locking the door behind me. The room was a typical patient room, but it was unclean, and the odor reflected that uncleanliness. At first, the patient came after me, swinging and landing occasionally, but since his only weapon was his body, I felt I could protect myself. My preparation for defending myself against violent attacks during the student sit-in movement came in handy. I had learned how to protect my face and head from punches and sticks. The young man swung hard, but he was not that strong, and after a few attempts, he tired out and we both sat down. We went through this on my first three visits with him. After he tired out and we both sat down, he began to talk. He wanted to know where I had learned to protect myself, so I told him about my experience growing up in Alabama in a family with six boys and two girls; how I survived the early illnesses in our home; and about the racial encounters in Alabama and Georgia. He was very interested, so we talked and talked.

This interaction helped to form a bond between us, so I gradually asked him about his thinking about race in general. He described how he often felt that he was being attacked by his own mind, hearing voices and seeing things, most of which he associated with race. I was able to convince him that he should take the medications the nurses brought to him two or three times a day, and he began to comply.

I reported back to my team on a regular basis, and the faculty used these reports to teach us about paranoid schizophrenia and medications that worked. I read everything the faculty assigned and more. I sought all that I could find on what this young man was going through.

My relationship with the patient continued; however, on one occasion, I had to be away from the rotation for almost a week. When I returned, the nurses told me that the patient was asking for me every day, and he often banged on the door and expressed fear that I was never coming back, and even that I had been harmed by the whites on the team. When I returned, he was elated and wanted to talk more and more.

The young man was never transferred to the state hospital, but continued to improve on his medical regimen and with our interaction. In time, his trust extended to the nurses and members on our team. After a few weeks, he was able to be discharged home on his medications. We promised to stay in contact. By knowing that young man I came to better understand the stigma that surrounds mental illness, and why people often associate it with violence. This was a special case where the illness involved an initial violent response in the context of race and interpersonal interactions. As the young man got better, I no longer saw him as a violent person, and in some ways he looked like a different person altogether. In retrospect, I could identify with the origin and nature of his paranoia. The reality of racial bias and discrimination certainly feeds this kind of paranoia. The fact that we had similar backgrounds and that I had been able to find a way to deal with them was real. So was this mental illness that made it more difficult for him to control his feelings. It was when I learned not to generalize racist behavior to "all white people" that I was better able to deal with the racism of some.

It is appropriate to ask again how leaders can work to reduce the stigma associated with mental illness. It is certainly one of the greatest challenges we face in health care. I believe that there are things that we can do to help reduce the stigma. First, and perhaps foremost, we can educate people in our communities about the nature of mental health and mental illness. Community mental health workers often do an exceptional job of community education and referral by emphasizing the prevalence of mental illness: perhaps as many as one in four Americans will experience some mental disorder or diagnosis each year.[28] Those who suffer with mental disorders are not alone, whether they are children, families, or adults. Discussing the fact that mental disorders are common, if emphasized appropriately, should help to reduce the stigma attached to them. We can also discuss the nature of mental disorders, making it clear that they are diseases of the brain. But demonstrating success in the treatment of mental disorders is most important.

There is too much of a cloud surrounding mental disorders, one that we believe could be lifted if more focus were put on the health of the brain and treatments that target different areas and functions of the brain. To emphasize that mental disorders are treatable, like any other illness, we can use examples of people who have shared their experience of treatment, such as Kay Redfield Jamison in her book *An Unquiet Mind*[29]—a book based on the author's bipolar disorder experience.

The fact that we are all at risk for mental disorders is important. Only by realizing our own risk do we gain the kind of empathy for others that may be missing. Just as things go wrong with the heart, the lungs, the kidneys, and the liver, things go wrong with the brain; they always have and they always will. Leaders need to emphasize that in words and by example. Jamison, a Johns Hopkins clinical psychologist, has continued, over the last thirty or more years, to write and speak and educate people all over the world about our ability to treat people with mental illness.

The gap between mental health and mental illness is often narrow, and none of us can take our mental health for granted. Indeed, one can be mentally healthy today and mentally ill tomorrow.

Social bias against individuals with mental illness puts all of us at risk. That so many people with mental disorders are in jails and prisons, as opposed to getting treatment in the appropriate facilities, should be of concern to all of us, and we should not wait until it impacts ourselves or our families. I am very pleased that an increasing number of judges are now sentencing patients with mental disorders to treatment programs instead of punishment. They sit at an important crossroads for these patients and show leadership in the way they wield their power. And yet, the punishment approach for persons with mental disorders is still all too common. Mental illness is treatable, and the earlier treatment begins, the more effective it is.

This is especially true of children with mental disorders. Children exist not just in families, but in a network of institutions: schools, church, the scouts, athletic teams, the community. Somehow, we need to conspire to make sure that children are supported in all of those settings, that when they have a mental health problem it is recognized early and treated as soon as possible. More than half of all mental disorders have onset before fourteen years of age,[30] which illustrates how important it is for us to target treatment to children and to begin early.

Finally, we must develop integrated teams to care for people with mental disorders. Such teams at a minimum must include primary care providers, mental health specialists, social workers, nurses, health educators, and when possible, community health workers. These teams must learn from each other as part of their training.

Integrated care is now a part of the strategy of the American Psychological Association for dealing with mental disorders.[31] It is clear that integrated care improves the quality of care for mental disorders; it improves access because it means that patients can often be helped in the primary care facility, where the diagnosis should be made. Our experience at Grady Hospital in Atlanta is one example of the impact that the integrated care approach can have upon patients and communities. However, in order for this approach to be implemented more broadly, training programs and support must be made available.

Stigma surrounding mental disorders is real; it is real for individuals, and it impacts them and their behavior, especially their help-seeking behavior. Stigma often interferes with families making decisions that are in the best interest of their children. It impacts communities, which often treat mental disorders as shameful instead of providing early diagnosis and needed care. Stigma also impacts policy makers and often leads either to care not being available or to care not being adequately funded. Often, policy makers have not required insurers to provide the kind of coverage that is available for other kinds of disorders. Therefore, policy makers are a part of the problem when it comes to the stigma surrounding mental disorders. Finally, and sadly, because of that stigma, health professionals often neglect the brain in the evaluation of patients, acting as if the brain were not a part of the overall body.

Leaders must take the responsibility for making sure that individuals, families, and the community are appropriately educated about the nature of mental disorders. In addition, leaders must work to develop the kind of environments where people with mental disorders are comfortable seeking care and can find support as opposed to abuse. We must educate and motivate the community to take the appropriate steps. We must continue to try and better understand the nature of stigma, and especially the way it relates to

culture. As more and more people become a part of the community, bringing their different histories, cultures, and backgrounds,
it is important to understand how that impacts the presence, man-
ifestation, and treatment of mental disorders.

Chapter Twelve

Leadership beyond Expertise

I N ORDER TO ACHIEVE health equity, we need leaders who first care enough, know enough, and have the courage to do enough, leaders who will persevere until the job is done. That may sound like an obvious statement, but it leads to some important questions, and it has become a motto at the leadership institute. But what does it mean to know enough? Clearly, no one person can be an expert in all the different areas necessary to achieve health equity. So how does one lead without being an expert?

On June 1, 2017, I received the Forsyth Icon Award for the Surgeon General's Report on oral health.[1,2] In my response, I revisited the report and updated some of its findings. But my training and background is in medicine and cellular biology, not in oral health. Of my reports, oral health is the one subject that could be considered farthest from my area of expertise.

As a rule, the Office of the Surgeon General maintains a list of potential topics for the development of new Surgeon General's Reports. Many topics will never be developed due to the time it takes to complete a report and the limited tenure, usually less than four years, of most surgeons general. But events such as the recent opioid addiction epidemic can certainly move a topic up the list rapidly.[3] Only once in my experience did the White House and Congress request a report with a specific topic. Soon after I was sworn in, the 1999 Columbine High School shootings occurred,[4] killing twelve students and one teacher. Such a mass shooting was a rare experience indeed in this country, or anywhere else at the time. The American people were shocked, and appropriately so. The request from the White House and Congress was that I develop a report on youth violence.

With the help of expertise, and some funding from the Substance Abuse and Mental Health Services Administration (SAMHSA) and the CDC,[5,6] I completed the report *Youth Violence Prevention*, in 2000.[7] As surgeon general, I coordinated the development of the report and led the communication about it. A special team at the CDC and at SAMHSA was assembled to complete the units of the report on violence, which expedited it and the report on oral health. They both had strong communications. Most of the expertise, however, came from the Injury Prevention Center at the CDC,[8] as well as the many experts in mental health and social science from SAMHSA, along with some private outside input. The oral health report was also assembled by a team led by Caswell A. Evans, DDS, MPH, Assistant Director, Los Angeles County Department of Health Services. The violence prevention report delayed the oral health report, but did not put it on hold.

When the report on violence was released, after approximately six months of intense work, the outcry of concern from the American people had abated, so the report did not get the attention and follow-through from Congress or the White House that we had anticipated. Also, the political implications of the topic of violence—especially involving guns and access to guns—probably prevented the kind of discussions by politicians that we had hoped for. Unfortunately, the issue is still alive, and the report is frequently referred to, but Congress has not acted on any policy that makes access to guns more difficult or mental health services more accessible.

Congressman Jay Dickey of Arkansas introduced legislation in 1996 to take funding from the CDC and use it to study the health-related impact of gun violence[9]—the research showed that possession of guns did not necessarily protect families. Instead, many families were put at risk for in-home violence, including suicide. Research on gun violence was gaining some momentum before the CDC Injury Prevention Center research funding was removed by Congress. Although the funding was less than $3 million, its loss has taken quite a toll on gun violence research. Shortly before his death on April 20, 2017, Congressman Dickey joined Dr. Mark Rosenberg, who had served as director of the Injury and Prevention Center while I was director of the CDC, in writing an op-ed piece in the *Washington Post*, asking that the money be restored to the CDC and research resumed on the issue of guns and violence.[10] Also, on January 14, 2016, Senator Dick Durbin of Illinois introduced legislation that would provide as much as $10 million of funding per year for the CDC to lead a deeper study and programmatic development for reducing gun violence.[11] The legislation did not pass, and this issue is still very much alive.

As the former surgeon general who had written *Youth Violence*, I was asked to lead the effort to put together a preliminary proposal. Even though my involvement is much less than when I served as director of the CDC, I'm still able to wield influence as a leader in the efforts to reduce violence in the United States. What do I bring to the table? I think at best, leaders assemble people with expertise and concerns around a particular issue, and coordinate the communication and collaboration of the group to reach a goal. The leader needs expertise on the bigger issues related to communication and policy and the assembly of expertise, but the leader's role is broader and must situate the issue in the context of the bigger picture.

After receiving all of the expert input into the Surgeon General's Report on oral health, we did two things that proved very useful. First, we developed and published an independent executive summary, describing the significance and content of the report, so that someone could sit down and in one reading completely understand the report's major findings and recommendations. It was the first such summary to be published in conjunction with a Surgeon General's Report. Interestingly enough, having seen how effective that format was, we later released the *Surgeon General's Call to Action to Prevent and Reduce Overweight and Obesity*,[12] which was basically an executive summary. It had a tremendous impact on the behavior of states and communities throughout the country, and on the way schools, as well as others, are approaching this problem. We brought together an interdisciplinary team of dentists, pediatricians, and related support personnel to approach oral health as the interdisciplinary field that it is. Oral health impacts the health of the whole individual, not just the mouth or teeth. The report from this meeting of the interdisciplinary team, in June of 2000, was called *The Face of a Child*.[13]

As surgeon general, I was credited with having communicated the report on oral health with clarity and passion. Since the office brings with it a level of authority, prestige, and trust, bringing the surgeon general's voice to an issue is in and of itself important for the success of such a report. Leadership at its best brings people together to deliberate the implication of scientific findings and the policy implications. Then leadership works to communicate clearly.

Leadership is always about clear and effective communication.

It is also about coordinating the expertise and commitment of a team. It's not always essential for a leader to be an expert, but leadership does rely on trust. The surgeon general communicates with authority and expertise that only comes with that level of involvement, coordination, and trust. That trust was begun with the first Surgeon General's Report, issued by Dr. Luther Terry in 1964, *Smoking and Health*.[14] Those of us who followed have tried to build upon it.

It is significant that before any report is released by the surgeon general, it must be signed off on by the top scientists at the CDC, the NIH, SAMHSA, and other relevant agencies. It is a cumbersome process, but when it is completed, the product is worthy of the kind of trust and authority that most reports from the surgeon general receive.

While it has lost most of the administrative authority it had when the surgeon general was also head of the Public Health Service,[15] the Office of the Surgeon General has grown as an independent source of information. That growth has been possible in part because the OSG is not a part of the administrative team, which must promote the positions, especially the political positions, of the White House, regardless of the science. The Surgeon General's Reports are based on the best available science, and not on politics. It is important to the American people when asked to "just say no" to smoking and drugs that solid science supports that advice.

I like to say that over the years the surgeon general has lost political power but gained authority and trust in communicating directly with the American people, based on the best available public health science. Since I served as both the assistant secretary for health and as surgeon general simultaneously, perhaps my experience best illustrates the difference. When I went to Washington in that dual capacity, in 1998, only one other person had served in both positions simultaneously. Dr. Julius Richmond served in both positions in President Carter's administration. Among other things,

Surgeon General Richmond released the report *Healthy People: The Surgeon General's Report on Health Promotion and Disease Prevention*,[16] which was the first to set goals and specific objectives to be achieved over the next decade. That report would become the model for future Healthy People reports, each aimed at a successive decade. For instance, Healthy People 2010 had its beginning in the year 2000, and it set objectives to be achieved by 2010.[17] The goals and their accompanying objectives, which involved people throughout the PHS,[18] probably represent the high point of my service as both surgeon general and assistant secretary for health.

I became the first CDC Director to be appointed to the position of surgeon general. The difficulty of holding both positions soon became clear. At the CDC, during the 1990s, we conducted thirty studies of the efficacy of the needles/syringes exchange program,[19] which was geared toward preventing the spread of HIV by drug users. The studies showed conclusively that these programs (1) prevented or greatly curtailed the spread of HIV, and (2) did not increase drug use, but resulted in many drug users getting into treatment programs.

Policy had not, however, caught up with the new science, so I asked the administration to request a policy adjustment from Congress to allow federal funding of the Needle Exchange Program. President Clinton was agreeable, and we scheduled a press conference to announce that the president would be asking Congress to change policy to adjust to the new science. We gathered the key experts together in a conference room in the Humphrey Building of the Department of Health and Human Services. However, less than an hour before this press conference, with the press already gathered outside of the room, we received a call from the White House telling us that the president had changed his mind and would not be asking Congress for this legislation. Among other things, we were told that the new drug czar had recommended against it. He felt that it would not pass Congress and would be used against the president in the upcoming election. Politically, I understood the concern, and as assistant secretary for health, I had to support the decision.

However, as surgeon general, my responsibility was to communicate and support science and a policy consistent with that science. I therefore communicated the results of our studies, and while they supported federal funding of needle exchange programs, why would we urge state funding of such programs? It felt somewhat schizophrenic, but it was clear to me and to others that my responsibility was to communicate on the basis of the best available science. It was the politics that would not allow the federal funding, not the science! I left that meeting, and as I traveled and interacted as surgeon general, I urged the funding of needle exchange programs. Many states did and still do support such programs. Today, as we write this, even the state of Georgia is developing support for needle exchange programs.

Long before I became a part of government, and before I dealt with the thousands of people I later oversaw at such a high level, I dealt with issues with which I personally lacked expertise. This can be a difficult situation, unless you have surrounded yourself with people whose expertise is superior to yours, and people whom you trust.

So, if leadership is not about expertise or knowing more about the subject matter than those you lead, how then does leadership relate to expertise? I would like to point to five very important areas of this relationship: leadership (1) *recognizes* expertise, (2) *respects* expertise, (3) *coordinates* expertise, (4) *encourages* expertise, and (5) *rewards* expertise.

Beyond that, a leader develops expertise that may or may not serve his or her leadership, but serves the future needs of institutions or organizations. People with expertise appreciate when their expertise is recognized. Sometimes this expertise is recognized by promotion of faculty, as in academia.

But academia is not alone having a system of promotion and recognition of expertise. If leaders fail to recognize and reward expertise, the institution or business suffers. Such recognition and respect require a certain level of security on the part of the leader. One has to be secure in his or her own areas of expertise to be comfortable recognizing publicly the expertise of others. Leaders who feel they must have expertise in all areas of institutional endeavors often suffer burnout or lose support.

Leadership must also manage expertise as a coach does in coaching a team. This means not only coordinating skills and training but also arranging the activity of experts who can sometimes find it difficult to work together. In order to carry out this function, the leader must be secure in his or her own self. Just as many coaches were not great athletes themselves, they have excelled in coordinating the expertise of outstanding players. When it works well, it is a winning team. Great expertise without great management falls flat on its face as far as the institution is concerned.

The leader may not meet with the experts on a regular basis, and may rely on members of the leadership team, such as vice presidents and department chairs. But quality coordination of expertise begins and ends with the leader. Just as with a basketball team, some players are best at controlling the ball and others at shooting it; the coach has to manage all of this. For example, the vice president for academic affairs meets with the various deans on a regular basis, whereas the president meets them much less often. In football, there is a coach for defense and one for offense, as well as for defensive linesmen and offensive linesmen.

Leadership must encourage expertise, because experts need and deserve to be encouraged at every level. It is, by the way, interesting how insecure some experts can be themselves with their expertise. The leadership team should involve all of the key areas of expertise: medicine, dentistry, graduate studies, and public health.

In the year 2000, as a part of Healthy People 2010, the Department of Health and Human Services proposed the elimination of disparities in health. I remember that when we were thinking about getting Congress to pass legislation to support this goal, Secretary Donna Shalala called me in for a discussion about the challenges we would face. Most important would be the funding of research needed to develop strategies for eliminating disparities in health. One of the most difficult challenges would be for our department (HHS) to speak with one voice. In government, as in academia, we don't tell people what to say when they make external presentations, including to Congress. Secretary Shalala was especially concerned that Nobel Laureate Dr. Harold Varmus,[20] who was director of the NIH at the time, might not be supportive of the specific legislation to support the goal and its implications for NIH. She thought it critical that I speak with Dr. Varmus, so he might come on board before he spoke to Congress at the budget hearing. Both the goal of eliminating disparities and the strategy/role of the NIH were tied together.

When I spoke to Dr. Varmus he indeed expressed concern about the goal of eliminating disparities in health and its implications for research carried out by the NIH and the people whom it funded. NIH did not have a record of funding many minorities in research, and saw no reason to change. In many ways they were resistant to goal-oriented research and to increasing minority representation in funding requests. The institute directors, such as Anthony Fauci, head of the AIDS Institute,[21] and Vivian Pinn, director of the Office of Research on Women's Health,[22] were outstanding experts in their fields. I anticipated that they would challenge our logic and plans. After our discussion about this, Harold called me and made a proposal. He wanted me to come to the quarterly meeting of the twenty-seven institute and center directors at NIH. There he wanted me to present the logic and reason behind the goal of eliminating disparities in health and the role of NIH in it.

As a rule, the institute and center directors at NIH, like Drs. Fauci and Pinn, were experts in every sense of the word. I knew Harold had come up with a well-conceived strategy to challenge my proposal and that I had to agree to come and meet with his NIH team of outstanding researchers. And, even though I had anxiety about it, I realized its importance and agreed to do it. Since the support of these institute leaders was critical to getting Congress to pass the legislation, I was indeed anxious. We could not afford to lose.

The goal of eliminating disparities in health was in jeopardy. First, it was clear that the NIH and the directors of its six centers and twenty-one institutes appreciated the opportunity to confront me directly. In a sense, their expertise was being recognized and engaged at the level of departmental and national leadership. To have any expectation that the goal would be adopted, we needed the support of this group, and we needed enthusiastic support.

It was quite an engaging meeting, as I made the presentation, responded to questions, and challenged the outstanding group of experts. Participants in this meeting still tell me how clearly they remember that meeting and how important it was for them. I made it clear that even though I felt very strongly about the goal of eliminating disparities in health, it would not be achieved unless NIH adopted it and worked to make it a reality. In short, I recognized the importance of their expertise and needed their support. Where they had doubt, I encouraged them that this was their time and that they could move our nation forward. I felt good after the meeting because the dialogue was rich; it was needed; and it had taken place. I proposed a special set-aside of funds to target disparities in health, and they resisted at first. I was pleasantly surprised at how attentive and respectful they were. It was as if they appreciated hearing their areas of expertise placed in the perspective of disparities in health. I tried to paint a picture in which they could see their areas of work but also how it intersected with other areas.

Relationships had been built that were critical for the future. After the meeting, Harold Varmus would write a very persuasive letter to Congress, urging the passage of the disparities legislation. In addition, he and I would co-author articles in scientific journals about the research implications of the goal of eliminating disparities in health. Attendees were challenged to provide new opportunities for young minorities to begin research careers and to spend time at NIH with support of NIH researchers. Questions were posed that needed to be targeted for funding. Gaps in research were identified that would help to close gaps in health care. At NIH, there were experts in CVD, Diabetes, HIV/AIDS, and neuroscience, to name a few. They all had implications for the goal of eliminating disparities in health.

While leaders may not excel in every area of expertise, it is important that they excel in communication and organization. Leaders must also clearly articulate the big picture and, as in our meetings, experts appreciate that.

Chapter Thirteen

The Team Approach to Leadership

L EADERSHIP IS A TEAM SPORT, and one of the first responsibilities of a leader is team building, with an ongoing responsibility for team development. The leader must manage
the leadership team, keeping in mind that the leader is not a savior
and that it is not just about the leader. Leaders must create the type
of environment that allows teams to develop and gel. Leaders must
see themselves in the context of history. Leaders and the leadership
team must be adequately prepared to not only follow the plan but
also respond to the unexpected.

Early in my tenure as a leader, I saw myself as a loner, and even
described leadership as a lonely road: The buck stops here. I remember when I was director of the Sickle Cell Research Center at
King/Drew Medical Center in Los Angeles, I had a very good staff,
from the library director to the program manager. They would often
talk among themselves about how a program project had to be "sat-

urated." It was a while before I realized that what they were saying was "Satcher-rated"—meaning that until I gave my approval, regardless of how well they thought they had done, the project was not finished. While in some ways this was a compliment, it separated me from the team in a way that was not always good.

Surely, leadership at its best is like a team sport, and it takes time and effort to build a successful team. Whether team members are inherited or recruited to their positions, they are the leader's team members, and the leader is responsible for how the team functions. Team members who are already in place when a leader comes on board could be valuable assets and should know that their experience is appreciated. But they must also realize that the new leader will build a new team, and to the extent that they are able to accept the newness of the team, the leader will be able to shape the team to fit his or her role.

At Meharry Medical College, I faced a significant challenge when I began my tenure in July 1982. There was a $25 million deficit owing to Meharry Hubbard Hospital caring for patients without reimbursement. Located in North Nashville, where the population was very poor, most patients could not or would not pay for their care, and so over the years the debt mounted. In 1981, the *New York Times* published an article projecting that Meharry Medical College would close.[1] Everybody acknowledged the value of the institution, which had graduated more than 50 percent of black physicians and dentists in America, an institution 75 percent of whose graduates went on to practice in underserved communities, rural and urban.

When I became president of Meharry, the person I chose as executive vice president had been at the institution for almost forty years. He was a legend. He had received Meharry's first NIH grant and had been a symbol of the pursuit of academic excellence. Together we developed what was called the plan for academic renewal, and we were able to get $5 million to support it from the Robert Wood Johnson Foundation,[2] a foundation that, during the feasibility study, had doubted Meharry's ability to raise $3 million. We ultimately raised a total of $38 million, with significant support from the Robert Wood Johnson Foundation.

C. W. Johnson found new energy for the struggle because he found new hope. Although he was there when I arrived, he became an active member of a new team, and we worked together to move the institution forward. I respected and appreciated him for what he had done, but especially for what he contributed to the plan for academic renewal. We fought some great battles together to the benefit of the institution. In time, we were able to pull Meharry out of the grips of closure and move forward with new strategies and new hope.

When leaders are insecure they fail to get the most from their team. Team building is a never-ending process; some people just will not fit into a new team with a new leader. The sooner this is clear, the better. One member of my team at Meharry, whom I had brought on, found it difficult to work with the team when he did not get his way. On one occasion, after the team had debated and agreed upon an approach to an issue, he still disagreed, and he took his disagreement to the board of trustees. Because I did not consider that good team play, I asked him to leave the team, and begrudgingly he did. I regretted having to take that action.

Diversity is an important characteristic of a leadership team, and the leader must understand and appreciate that diversity. Diversity provides several important ingredients for a successful team. First, no one leader can be expected to be an expert in all areas of institutional needs, especially when they include teaching, patient care, research, and community relations. A good leadership team is far more than the sum of its parts, because when it is properly managed, including the management of team relationships, it becomes a significant force. The book *Workplace Diversity*,[3] published in 1995, discusses the values of diversity. The authors outline the types and major impacts of diversity. There is, of course, the legal civil rights issue, and working toward diversity is important for compliance with the law. Furthermore, a diverse input makes for a better product. Another benefit of diversity is the impact that it has on the environment. Not only does diversity enrich the workplace for the team but it also provides access to a diverse group of stakeholders, whether they be consumers, purchasers of goods, students, faculty, or advocates.

Sometimes, the leadership team has to focus on itself, and it helps to get away from the institution or the business and concentrate on getting to know one another better in a casual environment, focusing on relationships and team functions. This does not necessarily require an agenda and should not be structured to the point that it takes away from the relaxing nature of what we call retreats.

When the team has discussed an issue and comes to an agreement, no one member of the team should seek to undermine the team. Every member should have an opportunity to give input to the team's discussion, but every member should not expect to have his or her way. By the same token, no board should encourage individual members of the team to break from the team on an issue, unless it is a matter of basic ethics and integrity. The leadership team is the leader's team as long as certain standards are adhered to.

In order for a leadership team to function optimally, each member must have individual access to the team leader. I tended to have leadership team meetings monthly and as needed, but I also had meetings with individual team members on a biweekly basis, or whenever they called to say they needed to see me. It is important for members of a leadership team to have easy access to the team leader, because they are sometimes expected to respond to urgent situations.

When we decided on the strategy, we decided to hold monthly family hours, to communicate to the entire Meharry Medical College family the nature of the strategy and the role that they could play in it. We expected our employees to understand what we were doing and to talk about it in the community; we even encouraged them to make certain announcements in their churches about what we were doing and why we were doing it. This meant that once a month, at the family hour, I would report for about fifteen to twenty minutes, and the rest of the time was open for questions and comments. There is some risk to this, and our board even questioned whether I should do it—whether leaders should ever put themselves in such a risky position. I felt that our status as an institution was at risk, and the only way forward was for me to take a risk. So we took the risk, which turned out to have been a good strategy, one that helped us to win what we called the battle of Nashville— getting the hospital board and the City Council to vote to merge Meharry Hubbard Hospital with the City Hospital, move the City Hospital to Meharry's campus, and invest $50 million upgrading Meharry Hubbard Hospital. In many ways it was a form of salvation for an institution that was on the brink of closing. Because of the family hours, two important things happened: (1) employees understood, and they strategically talked it up in the community, including in their churches, and (2) Meharry Medical College employees attended City Council meetings and expressed their support for the merger. Perhaps more than anything else, this was responsible for our success. As an institution, we virtually spoke with one voice in the community about what we were doing, why we were doing it, and why this was best for the City of Nashville.

Team play is critical, and leaders must see themselves as a member of the team. Good team leadership requires a level of humility because the leader must first acknowledge that he or she is not an expert in all areas of endeavor and therefore depends upon members of the team and their expertise to help lead the institution or organization forward. There is a level of pride that goes with good team play, and that level of pride moves institutions and organizations forward.

It is important to point out that the concept of functioning as a team is not limited to sports teams. It is certainly not like football, where most players have careers of less than three years. It is first a group of people with diverse talents brought together for a common purpose. It is also a dynamic group, in which people often move up and down the leadership ladder. In fact, it is this deep nature that helps to hold the team together over time—as it is enriched by success and shares mutually in the benefits of that success.

The team approach to leadership brings the leadership closer to the workers or members in the field. It thus enriches the workers in the field and adds to their feeling of engagement with major institutional issues. The team approach should enhance communication between top leadership and those in the field of activity. The CDC consists of centers and institutes, focusing on infectious diseases, HIV, and chronic conditions, such as hypertension, reproductive health, and adolescent health. Although these divisions changed from time to time with new leadership, as a rule these areas of expertise formed the basis for the CDC organization.

Each area of expertise had its own leadership, and these leaders were members of the CDC director's leadership team. There were two major advantages to this type of organization: first, it was intentionally enticing for those in various areas of expertise to work together and communicate with one another. Having a division leader who served as a member of the director's leadership team greatly enhanced the two-way flow of information. Knowing that the division or group leader was in close contact with the institute leader helped to reassure the group that their input was being heard and that information was flowing from the leader back to them on a regular basis. It also assured the top leader that his or her message was getting to the leaders in the various areas of expertise and that their reactions were getting back to him or her.

As I stated earlier, diversity is important for the relevant and productive function of an organization, but diversity only works if the leadership team is diverse. Decisions made at the top must have the benefit of diverse input and reaction to the top-level deliberation, and decisions must be based on a diversity of culture, background, and expertise. Properly managed, the top leader benefits tremendously from a leadership team that is diverse, and the overall workforce benefits from a leadership team that is diverse, thus assuring diverse input to top deliberations and decision making.

It is not easy to achieve optimal diversity on the leadership team, but it is certainly a goal that should be constantly sought. Sometimes, organizing advisory groups for frequent interaction with the leader or leadership team can help to achieve the goal of diverse input, but it must not be considered equivalent to a diverse leadership team.

So, if a team approach to leadership is not the same as leadership as a team sport, then how and why is it different? First, a leadership team is formed to provide leadership that is diverse and that supports top leadership. It is expected to provide expert input to top leadership in decision making and to manage those who will communicate the plans and decisions of the top leadership.

Members of the leadership team are chosen for their expertise, on the one hand, but also for their ability to lead and to work as members of a leadership team, on the other. In short, a leadership team is made up of leaders who also bring subject matter expertise. These leaders may not be the top experts in their field, but they have expertise in the field and they have leadership skills. They may not carry out the functions in their field of expertise, but they lead a group of people who carry out these functions.

How then does the leadership team function? The leadership team functions as a team that ultimately provides input to the top leader based on their area of expertise. This input may or may not have received the input of other people in the area of expertise, though ideally it should. Members of the leadership team understand and accept that the final decision comes from the top leaders and, ultimately, the board. But they have the opportunity to inform and influence other members of the leadership team, as well as the top team level. The ability to lead by influencing other members of the team and ultimately the top leader is an important leadership skill for members of the leadership team.

What happens when the leadership team is dealing with an issue that falls under the purview of one member of the leadership team, but there is disagreement about how the team should move forward? Again, sometimes an example serves best to make the point. On one occasion during my presidency at Meharry we were leading with a very tight budget, but we took seriously our need to balance our budget. In fact, our ability to raise funds was greatly enhanced because we were operating in the black. One year, we were close to balancing our budget, but not quite there. Then we realized that student tuition had not been raised in a few years, although other schools were consistently raising their tuition. Our associate dean for Student Affairs felt it was his responsibility to "look out" for the students, so he argued against raising tuition. The consensus was that if we raised tuition, no students would have to drop out; they would have a slightly higher debt when they entered practice, but they could afford to repay it. On the other hand, lack of a balanced budget could threaten our accreditation and certainly hurt our overall fund-raising. The consensus of the leadership team was that we should move forward and raise tuition. However, the dean held firmly to his opinion.

While I regretted our inability to reach total consensus, I respected the dean's position of protecting the students. When the board of trustees met, I was surprised when the dean spoke against our proposal to raise tuition as a strategy for balancing the budget. I thought we had made the decision as a leadership team to raise tuition levels, even though the decision was not unanimous. In short, I felt that the dean disrespected me, as president, and the leadership team by speaking out against our proposal before the board. The board was caught off guard, but in the end, decided to support my recommendation to increase tuition. It was awkward and somewhat embarrassing, but the decision was made for us to move forward.

What happens when one member of the leadership team decides to buck the team and the top leader and tries to get the board to go in a different direction? Certainly, it hurts the credibility of the leadership team and of the president. Fortunately, our board realized the danger we faced in terms of leadership credibility and acted appropriately. Unfortunately, I felt that it was my responsibility to act immediately and replace the dean. It was painful because he was a friend of mine, but I felt that, for the sake of the integrity of the leadership team, I had no choice. Failure of a member of the leadership team to persuade the team regarding a decision in his arena has to stop at that level. "The buck stops here" applies to a decision made by the leadership team. The failure of the dean to convince me and the other members of the leadership team that we should not raise tuition was a failure that had to be accepted, no matter how painful.

The leadership team approach actually gave workers in the field virtually direct contact or input to the top leaders. But, as stated earlier, I went further and started the so-called family hour at Meharry and the director's hour at the CDC. In both cases, these meetings, held monthly or every two months, were well attended. At the CDC, my administrative team recommended that we give the extended team the opportunity to submit questions ahead of time so that we could be sure to cover them. This worked well inasmuch as 30 percent of the CDC workforce worked from home, using online technology.

In sum, the team approach to leadership should greatly enhance communication at every level, allowing for a diversity of input that is increasingly desirable. I would agree with those who have written that team sports is not a good model for team leadership.[4] As a rule, team ownership and leadership generally rest with one person; whereas the team members or players might be a diverse group, the team leadership is generally fairly narrow. Players are usually paid well, especially in professional sports, but they have little or no authority when it comes to leadership of the team. They are not in a position to make the sport safer. They are in competition with one another to "make the team," even at great risk to their own health and future. They are in competition with other players to maintain their position. They have very little security beyond their playing years, and their future health has become a major issue in recent years, with the diagnoses of chronic traumatic encephalopathy (CTE) in many cases upon examination of brains of former players. There are certainly different kinds of teams, but not all of them can serve as a model for the team approach to leadership.

My last leadership position/role before developing SHLI/MSM was the interim presidency at the Morehouse School of Medicine. I had come to the MSM to develop the National Center of Primary Care and in support of its president. When he left, I was asked by the board to take over. Initially, I said no because I had made it clear when leaving government that I did not want to serve as president of an academic institution after having served in that role for almost twelve years at Meharry Medical College. But after both the board and the Faculty Senate prevailed upon me, I agreed to serve for six months, until a new president could be selected. It took almost two years and it was quite an enlightening experience. As never before,

I felt the need to work with the leadership team collectively and individually to strengthen leadership capacity at the institution.

We decided to develop and implement a leadership development strategy. Selfishly, I wanted to make certain others on the team would be prepared to assume the leadership roles. We examined leadership as a concept; we discussed leadership styles and strategies; and we read books written by some great leaders, such as John Maxwell,[5] Stephen Covey,[6] James Collins,[7] and Walter Fluker.[8] We discussed their concerns about assuming leadership roles, and together we made progress during the interim period. We set fundraising records with alumni and doubled the endowment while continuing academic growth.

For the first time in my leadership career, I took time to develop and enhance the leadership team. In part, it helped that I was secure in my leadership role and was comfortable turning it over to someone else when the time came. In retrospect, I believe that one of the key roles of the leadership team should be to develop the leadership skills of individual leaders and to grow as a team. Although leaders are often too stressed and insecure to play the role as it should be played, they can and should set aside time for team and individual leadership development. Retreats led by consultants who specialize in leadership development are probably the next best thing and should be encouraged.

When the new president arrived, I asked him and the board to allow the interim director of the National Center for Primary Care to stay on as director. I wanted to continue to work with leadership development in a more organized fashion. So the board voted for the establishment of the Satcher Health Leadership Institute in 2006. Details as to how the SHLI/MSM would be developed, how it would be funded, and even how it would function were not yet clear to the board or even to me. But I felt comfortable that it could work and that I would enjoy and make a contribution in making it work.

Chapter Fourteen

Leading for Institutional Sustainability

L EADERS MUST THINK beyond today for the long-term survival and growth of their institutions. Mission-oriented leaders must also have a clear vision about the institution's future, and build toward that future. For example, the mission of the Satcher Health Leadership Institute at Morehouse School of Medicine (SHLI/MSM) is *to develop a diverse group of leaders who are committed to the reduction and ultimate elimination of disparities in health*; its vision, *to be a transformative force in the quest for global health equity*, looks to the future. Viewing leadership in terms of the future is a statement of commitment to sustainability.

I offer the following example of sustainability: until recently, I had always been an avid runner. I was a long-distance runner in college in the 1960s, and in 2001, while serving as the surgeon general, I ran the Marine Corps marathon.[1] I tend to see life and leadership in terms of a long-distance run. In order to survive and thrive in a race, you must first develop a durable yet comfortable stride, you must be clear about the distance, and you must not burn energy unnecessarily. At the same time, you must maintain a competitive pace that allows you to accelerate in response to opportunities and challenges that may present themselves. Sometimes that even requires sprinting.

Unfortunately, crisis situations far too often create environments where leadership changes are made without consideration of the importance of continuity of relationships and efforts. This presents challenges for leadership boards, which are responsible for providing transitions that keep their institutions moving forward. Therefore, leadership boards must have a clear vision for the future of their institutions. Leading for the long term includes doing at least the following three things well:

1. *Continuing to build institutional resources*, including financial resources, in terms of budgetary funds and endowment, and human resources, in terms of the quality of faculty and staff, when appropriate. Fund-raising is clearly a part of the stability of an institution, but building an endowment is critical for the long term. However, investing in people is just as important, if not more so. Getting the right people on board goes a long way toward ensuring the sustainability of any institution.

2. *Leading for the long term includes continuing to develop a reputation for excellence and integrity.* The extent to which people are willing to support and invest in an institution is closely related to its reputation. Over time, institutions, like individuals, develop reputations. Being committed to excellence is a characteristic that allows donors to be comfortable that their awards will be wisely invested for the future and used appropriately.

   Developing a reputation for integrity is equally important— a reputation that says you are who you claim to be, and you can be trusted to do what you say you are going to do. There is no substitute for personal integrity, and that includes institutional integrity, which inspires people to offer their support and partnership.

3. *Leading for sustainability includes developing sustainable partnerships with those who share our missions and goals.* Developing sustainable partnerships can be more valuable than money in moving institutions forward. The SHLI/MSM has been very fortunate to have partnerships that have enabled its fellows and students to participate in programs that it could not finance. Sustainable partnerships enrich our programs, provide shared resources, and allow us to look to the future with colleagues who have similar missions and goals.

Leaders must model sustainability in their lives and behavior. This includes practicing physical, mental, social, and spiritual renewal. Successful leaders must continually renew themselves by planning for periods away to reflect. My family and I generally took a three-week vacation every year, and I always returned to work with renewed energy, fresh ideas, and more determination.

I learned that many of my faculty and staff did not take a vacation. Unused vacation hours showed up on the institution's balance sheet as a deficit. A new strategy, whereby employees were given a specific period of time to use or lose their accumulated time, was approved by the board of trustees. The institution benefitted financially and otherwise by having rejuvenated employees. I think personal rejuvenation must be a part of any plan to maximize performance.

We must sustain ourselves in order to sustain our institutions. Productive workers at every level play an important role in sustaining an organization. Ultimately, each of us must renew ourselves on a daily basis. I attempt to set aside two hours each morning for physical activity, meditation, and other strategies for renewing my mind. I strongly recommend this as a component of personal sustainability. Finally, leaders must plan for and look to the future in everything that they do because their role is to sustain the institution, even through a change of leadership.

Since it was established in 2006, in keeping with its three-dimensional approach to sustainability, the SHLI/MSM has developed a reputation for *integrity and excellence, strong and enduring partnerships, and a base of productive resources, especially endowment or long-term committed funding.*

What happens to the sustainability of an institution when the environment that caters to its development changes and its role and the need for it change? This is the issue that many historically black colleges and universities, black organizations, and institutions have faced over the last half century and continue to face today.

Near the end of the nineteenth century, predominantly black organizations and institutions were developed so that black students and professionals would be able to learn and develop their skills in the face of exclusion by predominantly white organizations and institutions. One example is the National Medical Association (NMA), founded in 1895 as an organization representing black physicians,[2] who, in most areas, were excluded from state and local chapters of the American Medical Association (AMA) during the period of segregation.[3] It was out of this exclusion and concern for its implications that the NMA was born, with leadership initially coming from graduates of the two historically black medical schools, Howard University and Meharry Medical College. These organizations were important for the camaraderie and continuing education of physicians. Convening to share information and motivation enhanced the knowledge, practice, and durability of attending physicians. In time, peer-reviewed publications, such as the *Journal of the American Medical Association (JAMA)*, came into being.[4]

The NMA thus played the role for black physicians that was denied them by the AMA and its local chapters. In time, the NMA convened its own national meetings and educational organization, as well as developing the *Journal of the National Medical Association* (*JNMA*).[5] At its annual meetings, the NMA provided programs for the sharing of information. A few of the members published articles from their experience in the field, as did faculty of Howard and Meharry.

The issue of sustainability became real as integration advanced in the twentieth century. Although black physicians were more likely to practice in black and underserved communities, they were, as a rule, no longer excluded from the AMA and its state and local chapters. Thus, the question about the need for the NMA was a growing issue, locally and nationally. Sustainability requires mission, and mission defines need.

It was thus the policy debate around access and care that helped to define the need and mission of the NMA and its chapters. The debate unfolded in the context of 1965 legislation to enhance access to care, by establishing two national programs: Medicare for the elderly and Medicaid for the poor.[6] As the debates advanced to the end of the 1960s, it helped to define the unique roles of the NMA and the AMA.

The AMA, the most powerful organization of physicians in America, opposed the creation of Medicare and Medicaid, even though more elderly participants were excluded from health access because they were no longer employed and insured and could not afford care. The AMA's expressed concern about government intervention in health care was understandable. Health care was viewed as a business, which should be left to doctors and patients without governmental interference. The NMA disagreed. Many of the patients did not have the ability to pay and required physician volunteers for sustenance. Thus, the two largest organizations of physicians in the United States took different sides on this critical issue. The NMA, established to assure that black physicians had an organization that supported their need for camaraderie and continuing education, became the voice of the elderly and the poor, and fought for the passage of Medicare and Medicaid. One might argue that the NMA was also fighting for its members, who often provided care without reimbursement.

When legislation establishing Medicare and Medicaid passed, it was clear that the mission of the NMA was broader than race. This legislation opened the door for President Lyndon B. Johnson and the secretary of Health, Education, and Welfare to speak at NMA's national meetings, and in time members of the NMA would rise to national leadership roles.

This was a turning point not only in the mission and status of the NMA but also in its sustainability. The need for and the role of the NMA were placed on solid ground, and it would never be the same. The AMA would begin to view the NMA as a collegial organization, and the president of the AMA would attend and speak at annual meetings of the NMA. By this same token, black physicians would become increasingly active in the AMA, holding dual memberships. Some white physicians now join the NMA and become active with its local and state chapters.

Thus, one might argue that in order to remain sustainable, organizations and institutions must respond uniquely to unmet needs. To the extent that those needs are met by others, the mission and sustainability of institutions are challenged. This is especially true when the others are both better funded from tax money or from private funds, including endowments.

The issue of sustainability is more complex when dealing with the role of HBCUs other than the two schools of medicine. Like Howard University and Meharry Medical College, most of the HBCUs were founded in the nineteenth century.[7] During this period, both private and state-funded universities often excluded black students, especially in the South; Northern schools rarely admitted black students, although they usually did not express a policy of segregation.

The battle to integrate or desegregate schools, including colleges, began to play out in the middle of the twentieth century. There were more than 100 HBCUs, both private and public, and most black college students attended one of these schools at that time. In the South, there was strong resistance by white, segregated schools and colleges to admitting black students. I remember this well from personal experience. I was bused almost twenty miles from my home outside of Anniston, Alabama, to the Calhoun County Training School in Hobson City, although there was a high school within two miles of my home! My younger siblings, Larry and Harry (twins), who were nine years my junior, would be in the first group of black students to attend Wellborn High School, the white school close to our home. Larry would graduate with honors, and Harry would be a leader in confronting the abuse they encountered.

When I was thirteen years old, candidate for governor George Wallace came through my hometown when he sought office a second time. He determined that he must show himself as a stronger segregationist than his opponent. While speaking in the park (also segregated), my brother Charlie hid with some friends and heard George Wallace promise that if he were elected governor, he would deputize every white man in Alabama before he would allow one black man to attend the University of Alabama. After his election, Governor Wallace would not be able to keep his promise; the University of Alabama accepted its first black student in 1963[8]—but the university's environment was hostile.

At the end of the 1950s, I applied to four HBCUs—Talladega College, Tuskegee Institute, Morehouse College, and Fisk University— all outstanding black colleges, but all segregated by history and law. As discussed earlier, after four years at Morehouse College, where I rose to leadership in the civil rights student movement,[9] I applied to medical school at Duke University, which had never accepted a black student into its undergraduate or graduate programs. Apparently, I was a finalist among two black applicants. Duke selected the other student, who had attended an integrated Michigan State University and had not been involved in the student movement.

Although I was deeply disappointed at not being a part of the integration at Duke University, I enrolled in the MD/PhD program at Western Reserve University, which probably led to what would be my success in medicine and other careers over the years. But I was deeply hurt when I was rejected by Duke, and even suffered some depression during my last months of college.

In the last half of the twentieth century, more and more black students were accepted into predominately white institutions in the South and throughout the United States. While this was generally good for black students, it meant that HBCUs had to compete for top black students. Thus, academic and financial sustainability became a growing concern for them by century's end.

A few years ago, the then president of Morehouse College explained to me the challenge of sustainability for one of the strongest historically black colleges—Morehouse. In 1959, when I enrolled at Morehouse, the college had its pick among outstanding, strong black students. Over 80 percent of Morehouse students had graduated in the top 10 percent of their high school classes. That has since changed to 80 percent of black students graduating in the top 10 percent of their high school class going to predominately white colleges. Many of the state schools are much more financially stable than we are. Thus, the struggle of HBCUs for sustainability is real and raises some key questions.

First, it is clear that not all HBCUs are equally sustainable, and it is highly likely that not all HBCUs will survive. While their missions may continue to be relevant, other institutions will adapt their missions to be more and more inclusive, not only of black students, but to meet the needs of those students and the communities from which they come and hopefully will return.

It is difficult to define the resource requirements for sustainability of an HBCU. For example, the endowments of educational institutions in the United States range widely from multiple billions to the low millions, and state-supported institutions are clearly not as dependent on endowments as others. As a rule, private HBCUs do not have the kind of endowments that historically white institutions take for granted, although the range of endowments for those institutions is quite wide. Today, only one HBCU has an endowment above $500 million—Howard University, with $685.8 million—followed by Spelman College, with $346.8 million.[10]

Upon examination of Meharry's financial situation, I became convinced that its financial crisis could be solved and its academic programs restored. With clarity in my own mind about what was required to regain Meharry's accreditation, I accepted the presidency in July 1982. It should be pointed out that Meharry's financial feasibility plan had been ruled negative. But along with the board and highly motivated staff, we developed a plan for academic renewal, which included raising $33 million over five years.[11] The story about how the Robert Wood Johnson Foundation contributed the first $5 million and provided other funds, helping to raise a total of $38 million, has already been told. Our accreditation was completely restored—and accreditation must be considered a prerequisite for sustainability. In Atlanta, Morris Brown College has remained open for sixteen years since the loss of its accreditation, with just a few students. It is fair to say that there is no defined level of funding required for sustainability. However, funding must be adequate to allow for accreditation. Accreditation often requires a strong faculty and student performance to demonstrate that high-quality education is taking place. Unlike the National Medical Association, whose members are licensed at the State level or certified by boards in their disciplines, HBCUs must be accredited in and of themselves, and not every college requires the same level or stages of faculty to assure the kind of student performance or achievement required for accreditation.

Some institutions are clearly able to do more in terms of education with fewer resources than other institutions. This may well relate to sustainability of faculty and programs over a long period of time. Leadership at the board, presidency, staff, and faculty levels seems to make a significant difference here.

Consistency of support from alumni is also critical for fundraising, recruitment of students, and board leadership. On the other hand, alumni can sometimes be obstructive to progress if they are not regular contributors, and even hold grudges based on their view of how they were treated as students.

Earlier, we discussed our experiences with alumni of Meharry Medical College when we made the decision to take alums to court if they were not repaying their institutional loans and thus threatening the validity of Meharry's student loan program. We regretted having to make such a decision, but it worked in the interest of present and future students. Alumni support in all forms is crucial for the sustainability of all institutions, especially HBCUs. Perhaps the most significant question, focusing on the sustainability of HBCUs, is the question of mission or need or unique purpose. Here is where I think we face the most important questions and indeed can make the strongest argument. Given students who, based on their credentials, are rejected by predominately white institutions, can we argue that HBCUs do a better job of preparing them for future careers? There is growing evidence that students chosen for medical schools with lower credentials often do better than expected on board exams and, in fact, in medical practice and careers. The American Association of Medical Colleges (AAMC) today is taking a close look at this issue and the associated data.[12]

The question is whether there is something about the environment and interaction of faculty and minority students that is more conducive to learning and performance at HBCUs. Clearly, the historically white state schools and universities have more resources to offer all of their students and are more affordable for most black students. But have we looked at their performance, not only at those schools, but also as they move forward for careers in medicine, law, and business, when compared with similar students at predominately black HBCUs?

Perhaps the basic issue relative to the sustainability of predominately black HBCUs is whether they still meet a unique need that is not being filled. Which institutions do the best? This question is not unrelated to the question of health equity. We define health equity not as health service equity, but as a system that provides persons with what they need, when and where they need it, in order to be healthy. When I entered Morehouse College in 1959, we faced a battery of tests during that first week of school. Because of my doubts about my ability to compete with most of the students— given my background in Anniston, Alabama, and with two parents who never finished elementary school—I had worked hard during the summer on my vocabulary, reading, math, and related areas, and I scored in the top 10 percent.

However, several of the students, most of whom had graduated in the top 10 percent of their high school classes, and even as valedictorians, did not do well on these tests and were placed in remedial classes. Many of the students who started taking remedial classes were able to catch up and graduate with honors and be accepted into medical, law, and other professional schools. Morehouse College tried to give them what they needed, when they needed it, in order to be successful not only at Morehouse but beyond.

We began this discussion of sustainability or challenge to lead for the long term with three areas of focus: (1) continuing to build institutional resources in the area of income and endowment, (2) continuing to develop a reputation for excellence and integrity, and (3) developing and maintaining sustainable partnerships. I have probably not, in the three areas, done justice to the role of mission in sustainability. To the extent that an institution is led to continue to speak to an unmet need that it clearly articulates, it will likely be sustainable.

To be clear, fund-raising and support is not successful because we have dire institutional needs that we articulate. It is successful because we have a mission that is clear and convincing, and to the extent that we have need, we have a plan to address that need, a plan that those with resources can feel comfortable helping us address. We begin with a vision for the future but must formulate a convincing plan to address our needs.

It is important for leaders to have a long-term perspective for the institution they lead, even though their leadership tenure may be limited. In most cases, the institution has been around long before its current leader, and it will need the resources and attitude to endure well into the future. Thus new leadership must plan for the continued existence of the institution by developing attitudes, resources, and a reputation that will serve the institution for many years.

In short, leadership must build for the long-term viability of the institution. Among the things the leadership must build are the *leadership team, a reputation for excellence, partnerships, endowment, and other lasting resources.*

New leadership must be comfortable with the mission of the institution and also have a vision for the institution's future. Such a vision must be shared not only with the leadership team but throughout the organization.

The vision of the World Health Organization, which accompanied the release of the SDH, is the ultimate achievement of global health equity. Before there was a clear approach and understanding of the role of these determinants, it was not possible to visualize the achievement of global health equity. But with an understanding and appreciation of them, the achievement of global health equity became a goal, a vision within reach of the global community. With this new vision, the global community has been able to define new sustainable goals. Within the context of a new vision and good leadership, institutions are able to redefine their missions and to set new goals.

In order for institutions to be sustainable, leadership must have these three very important properties of public health: *perspective, preparation, and partnership.*

Perspective is the context in which one sees the world. The wrong perspective can lead to the wrong interpretation of problems that need to be solved. On my trip to Malawi in 1986 to visit with President Banda, a physician and graduate of Meharry Medical College, I brought with me a limited perspective. I knew that teenage pregnancy was a problem in the United States, but I didn't understand why, in Africa, it was not seen as a problem. Only when I came to understand the plight of women in most of Africa did I realize the magnitude of the issue and problem. At that time, women in Africa were generally not allowed to go beyond elementary school, and many young girls would marry before they became adults and would often be one of many wives to a man.

Among other things, in the midst of the HIV/AIDS epidemic, one man would often be responsible for infecting several women with the virus. This led UNICEF to disclose to me that the most significant intervention to reduce the spread of HIV/AIDS in Africa would be the education of women.[13] This new perspective has done much to reduce the spread of AIDS in Africa and is a major component of a treatment strategy (PEPFAR),[14] which also significantly reduces the spread of the virus.

Without the right perspective, it is difficult to lead locally and globally. The right strategy begins with the right perspective.

The right *preparation* is required for strong effective leadership. In 1996, when I served as director of the CDC, we set a goal of eliminating polio in the world by 2001. India had more cases of polio than any other country, so we targeted India. We sent an outstanding team to prepare for a major push there—a push that would include the immunization of 100 million children in one week. My role was to join the team near the end of this effort. We had the support of Rotary International: 57,000 Rotarians came out to help get children to immunization sites.[15] We were well-prepared, and after three to four of these types of effort, we were able to eliminate polio in India.

India and our polio elimination effort there exhibited two very important examples of preparation and partnership. I can think of no better partnership than that between the CDC and Rotary International. We eliminated polio in India by 2011, but continue to struggle with our effort in Nigeria, Pakistan, and Afghanistan, mainly because of war efforts in those countries, especially the last two. The fighting in Afghanistan, Pakistan, and Nigeria make it difficult to get vaccine to children in those countries. But we are very close to eradicating polio in the world.

So whether our goal is to sustain an organization, an institution, or a disease-free status, we will need the right perspective, preparation, and we will need key *partnerships*. Thus, the sustainability of HBCUs depends on having the right perspective, preparation, and partnership.

ACA: Affordable Care Act

CDC: Centers for Disease Control and Prevention

CSDH: Commission on Social Determinants of Health

HBCU: historically black colleges and universities

HHS: US Department of Health and Human Services

IOM: Institute of Medicine

MMC: Meharry Medical College

MSM: Morehouse School of Medicine

NIH: National Institutes of Health

OSG: Office of the Surgeon General

PHS: Public Health Service

SAMHSA: Substance Abuse and Mental Health Services Administration

SDH: Social Determinants of Health

SHLI/MSM: Satcher Health Leadership Institute at Morehouse School of Medicine

References

INTRODUCTION

1. United States Census Bureau. *Census of Population and Housing*. Available from http://www.census.gov/prod/www/decennial.html.

2. Sprayberry, G. Anniston. *Encyclopedia of Alabama*, February 14, 2008. Available from http://www.encyclopediaofalabama.org/article/h-1464.

3. History.com. (2009; updated 2019). Civil Rights Movement. *A+E Network*. Available from http:www.history.com/topics/black-history/civil-rights-movement.

4. Ushistory.org. (2016). The Sit-In Movement. *US History Online Textbook*. Available from http://www./us/54d.asp.

5. Children's Defense Fund. A Strong, Effective, Independent Voice for All the Children of America. Available from http://www.childrensdefense.org/?referrer=https://www.google.com/.

6. "The Greatest Black Preachers," *Ebony*, September 1984, ISSN 0012-9011, p. 30. Available from https://books.google.com/books?id=DzMzhOLmewC&q=greatest+black+preachers#v=snippet&q=greatest%20black%20preachers&f=false.

7. Goodreads. Benjamin E. Mays Quotes. Available from http://www.goodreads.com/quotes/3235-it-must-be-borne-in-mind-that-the-tragedy-of.

8. Undelivered Remarks for Democratic State Committee, Municipal Auditorium, Austin, Texas, November 22, 1963. John F. Kennedy Presidential Library and Museum. Available from https://www.jfklibrary.org/Asset-Viewer/Archives/JFKPOF-048-023.aspx.

9. Learn about the Affordable Care Act. Available from http://hhs.gov/health care/about-the-aca/index.html/.

10. Impact of the Quality Parenting / Smart and Secure Children Parent Leadership Program. Available from http://satcherinstitute.org/division-of -behavioral-health/smart-and-secure-parenting-leadership-program/.

11. US Department of Health and Human Services, Office of the Surgeon General, Office of Population Affairs. *The Surgeon General's Call to Action to Promote Sexual Health and Responsible Sexual Behavior.* Rockville, MD: OSG, July 2001. Available from US GPO, Washington, DC.

CHAPTER 1. LESSONS LEARNED FROM FIFTY YEARS OF LEADERSHIP

1. Collins, J. C. (2001). *Good to Great: Why Some Companies Make the Leap . . . and Others Don't.* New York: Harper Business.

2. History.com. (2009; updated 2019). Civil Rights Movement. *A+E Network.* Available from http:www.history.com/topics/black-history/civil-rights -movement.

3. Ushistory.org. (2016). The Sit-In Movement. *US History Online Textbook.* Available from http://www.ushi.story.org/us/54d.asp.

4. Civil Rights Movement Veterans: An Appeal for Human Rights. March 9, 1960. Available from http://www.crmvet.org/docs/aa4hr.htm.

5. US Centers for Medicare and Medicaid Services. What's Medicare and Medicaid? Available from https://www.medicare.gov/Pubs/pdf/11306-Medicare -Medicaid.pdf.

6. "Meharry Medical College Is Troubled by Deepening Financial Crisis." *New York Times News Summary.* March 4, 1981. A12, 4–6. Available from http:// www.nytimes.com/1981/03/04/nyregion/news-summary-wednesday-march-4 -1982.html.

7. Johnson, C. W. (2000). *The Spirit of a Place called Meharry: The Strength of Its Past to Shape the Future.* Franklin, TN: Hillsboro Press.

8. Centers for Disease Control and Prevention. Available from http://www .cdc.gov.

9. Shands, K. N., G. P. Schmid, B. B. Dan, D. Blum, R. J. Guidotti, N. T. Hargrett, R. L. Anderson, et al. (1980). "Toxic Shock Syndrome in Menstruating Women: Association with Tampon Use and Staphylococcus aureus and Clinical Features in 52 Cases." *N Engl J Med* 303, no.25: 1436–1442.

10. Centers for Disease Control and Prevention. (December 22, 2006). "Behavioral and Social Sciences and Public Health at CDC." *Morbidity and Mortality Weekly Reports* 55 (SU02): 14–16. Available from http://www.cdc.gov /mmwr/preview/mmwrhtml/su5502a6.htm.

11. Office of Disease Prevention and Health Promotion. Healthy People. Available from https://health.gov/our-work/healthy-people/.

12. Satcher, D. Keynote Address to the American Pharmaceutical Association. Washington, DC., March 13, 2000.

13. US Department of Health and Human Services. *Mental Health: A Report of the Surgeon General.* Rockville, MD: HHS, Substance Abuse and Mental Health Services Administration, Center for Mental Health Services, National Institutes of Health, National Institute of Mental Health, 1999.

14. US Department of Health and Human Services. *Oral Health in America: A Report of the Surgeon General.* Rockville, MD: HHS, National Institute of Dental and Craniofacial Research, National Institutes of Health, 2000.

15. US Department of Health and Human Services. *The Surgeon General's Call to Action to Prevent and Decrease Overweight and Obesity.* Rockville, MD: HHS, Public Health Service, Office of the Surgeon General, July 2001.

CHAPTER 2. FROM HEALTH DISPARITIES TO GLOBAL HEALTH EQUITY

1. Centers for Disease Control and Prevention. Community Health and Program Services. *Health Disparities among Racial/Ethnic Populations.* Atlanta, GA: US Department of Health and Human Services, 2008. Available from https://www.cdc.gov/healthyyouth/disparities/.

2. National Institutes of Health. US National Library of Medicine. Health Services Research Information Central. 2009 Medical Subject Headings. Available from https://www.nlm.nih.gov/hsrinfo/disparities.html.

3. Nelson, A. (2002). "Unequal Treatment: Confronting Racial and Ethnic Disparities in Health Care." *Journal of the National Medical Association* 94 (8): 666.

4. Marwick, C. (2000). "Healthy People 2010 Initiative Launched." *JAMA* 283 (8): 989–990. doi:10.1001/jama.283.8.989. Available from http://jamanetwork.com/journals/jama/article-abstract/192422.

5. Fielding, J. E., S. Teutsch, and H. Koh. (2012). "Health Reform and Healthy People Initiative." *American Journal of Public Health* 102 (1): 30–33. doi:10.2105/AJPH.2011.300312. Available from http://ajph.aphapublications.org/doi/abs/10.2105/AJPH.2011.300312.

6. National Center for Health Statistics. *Healthy People 2000 Final Review.* Hyattsville, MD: Public Health Service, 2001. Available from https://www.cdc.gov/nchs/data/hp2000/hp2k01.pdf.

7. US Department of Health and Human Services. *Healthy People 2010.* Washington, DC: HHS, January, 2000. Available from www.health.gov/healthy people/.

8. US Department of Health and Human Services. *The NIH Almanac.* National Institute on Minority Health and Health Disparities. Bethesda, MD: HHS. Available from https://www.nih.gov/about-nih/what-we-do/nih-almanac /national-institute-minority-health-health-disparities-nimhd.

9. US Department of Health and Human Services. *Racial and Ethnic Approaches to Mental Health.* Atlanta, GA: Centers for Disease Control and Prevention. Available from https://www.cdc.gov/nccdphp/dnpao/state-local-programs/reach/.

10. MacDorman, M. F., and T. J. Mathews. "Understanding Racial and Ethnic Disparities in U.S. Infant Mortality Rates." *NCHS Data Brief,* no 74. Hyattsville, MD: National Center for Health Statistics, 2011. Available from https://www .cdc.gov/nchs/data/databriefs/db74.pdf.

11. Satcher, D., G. E. Fryer, J. McCann, A. Troutman, S. H. Woolf, and G. Rust (2005). "What If We Were Equal? A Comparison of the Black-White Mortality Gap in 1960 and 2000." *Health Affairs* 24: 459–464.

12. Arias, E. (2003). United States Life Tables. *National Vital Statistics Reports* 54 (4). Available from https://www.cdc.gov/nchs/data/nvsr/nvsr54/nvsr54_14.pdf.

13. Fryer, R. G., P. S. Heaton, S. D. Levitt, and K. M. Murphy. (2005). *Measuring the Impact of Crack Cocaine* (No. w11318). National Bureau of Economic Research. Available from http://www.nber.org/papers/w11318.pdf.

14. Evans, W., C. Garthwaite, and T. J. Moore. (2015). The White/Black Educational Gap, Stalled Progress, and the Long-Term Consequences of the Emergence of Crack Cocaine Markets. Available from http://www.kellogg.north western.edu/faculty/garthwaite/htm/Education_Crack.pdf.

15. Commission on Social Determinants of Health. *Closing the Gap in a Generation: Health Equity through Action on the Social Determinants of Health.* Final report of the CSDH. Geneva: World Health Organization, 2008.

16. McGinnis, J. M., and W. H. Foege. (1993). "Actual Causes of Death in the United States." *JAMA* 270 (18): 2207–2212. doi:10.1001/jama.1993 .03510180077038. Available from http://jamanetwork.com/journals/jama /article-abstract/409171.

17. US Department of Health and Human Services. *Physical Activity and Health: A Report of the Surgeon General.* Atlanta, GA: HHS, Centers for Disease Control and Prevention, National Center for Chronic Disease Prevention and Health Promotion, 1996.

18. Satcher, D. Keynote Address to the American Pharmaceutical Association. Washington, DC, March 13, 2000.

19. Tovrov, D. (2011). "5 Biggest Slums in the World." *International Business Times.* Available from http://www.ibtimes.com/5-biggest-slums-world-381338.

20. History.com. Hurricane Katrina. (2009). *A+E Networks*. Available from http://www.history.com/topics/hurricane-katrina.

21. Whoriskey, P. (2007). "Hurricane Katrina Exacts Another Toll: Enduring Depression. *Washington Post*, Sept. 23. Available from http://www.washington post.com/wp-dyn/content/article/2007/09/22/AR2007092200600.html.

22. CDC/National Center for Health Statistics. *Healthy People 2020*. Available from https://www.cdc.gov/nchs/healthy_people/hp2020.htm.

23. H.R. 3590: Patient Protection and Affordable Care Act. 111th Congress, 2009–2010. Public Law No: 111-148. March 23, 2010. Available from https://www.congress.gov/bill/111th-congress/house-bill/3590.

24. Centers for Medicare and Medicaid Services. The Center for Consumer Information and Insurance Oversight. The Mental Health Parity and Addiction Equity Act of 2008. Baltimore, MD. Available from https://www.cms.gov/cciio/programs-and-initiatives/other-insurance-protections/mhpaea_factsheet.html.

Chapter 3. When Leadership Confronts Failure

1. Charles R. Drew Website. Available from https://www.cdrewu.edu/.

2. Meharry Medical College Website Quick Facts. Available from https://www.mmc.edu/_modules/events/didyouknow2.html.

3. "Meharry Medical College Is Troubled by Deepening Financial Crisis." *New York Times News Summary*. March 4, 1981. A12, 4–6. Available from http://www.nytimes.com/1981/03/04/nyregion/news-summary-wednesday-march-4-1981.html.

4. Ushistory.org. (2016). The Sit-In Movement. *US History Online Textbook*. Available from http://www.ushi.story.org/us/54d.asp.

5. Schuller, R. H. (1988). *Success Is Never-ending, Failure Is Never Final*. Nashville, TN: Thomas Nelson.

6. "There are none so blind as those who will not see." Available from http://www.actualfreedom.com.au/richard/abditorium/nonesoblind.htm.

Chapter 4. The Need for Clear Communication

1. History.com. (2010). Montgomery Bus Boycott. *A+E Networks*. Available from http://www.history.com/topics/blackhistory/Montgomery-bus-boycott.

2. Ushistory.org. (2016). The Sit-In Movement. *US History Online Textbook*. Available from http://www.ushi.story.org/us/54d.asp.

3. Trueman, C. N. (2015). "Bull Connor." *The History Learning Site*, March 27. Available from http://www.historylearningsite.co.uk/the-civil-rights-movement-in-america-1945-to-1968/bull-connor/.

4. History.com. (2010). Civil Rights Act. *A+E Networks*. Available from http://www.history.com/topics/black-history/civil-rights-act.

5. US Department of Justice. History of Federal Voting Rights Laws. Available from https://www.justice.gov/crt/history-federal-voting-rights-laws.

6. Goodreads. Ernest Hemingway Quotes. Available from http://www.goodreads.com/quotes/353013-i-like-to-listen-i-have-learned-a-great-deal.

7. Active Listening. Business Dictionary.com. WebFinance, Inc. Available from http://www.businessdictionary.com/definition/active-listening.html.

8. Reference. What Are Some Examples of Passive Listening? Available from https://www.reference.com/world-view/examples-passive-listening-f9fad8c8699 ae55b?qo=cdpArticlesReference.com.

9. Intrator, D. "Creativity and Listening." The Creative Organization: Education for 21st Century Success. June 22, 2011. Available from http://the creativeorganization.com/creativity-and-listening/.

10. Goodreads. Theodore Roosevelt Quotes. Available from http://www.goodreads.com/quotes/34690-people-don-t-care-how-much-you-know-until -they-know.

11. Fagan, B. (2016). Aggressive Listening. The A Position: Where You Want to Land. Available from http://theaposition.com/robertfagan/coaching/life -coaching/2717/aggressive-listening.

12. Johnson, C. W. (2000). *The Spirit of a Place Called Meharry: The Strength of Its Past to Shape the Future*. Franklin, TN: Hillsboro Press.

13. Goodreads. Benjamin E. Mays Quotes. Available from http://www.goodreads.com/quotes/3235-it-must-be-borne-in-mind-that-the-tragedy-of.

14. King, M. L., Jr. (1963). "I Have a Dream." Speech. Lincoln Memorial, Washington, DC. August 28. Available from https://www.archives.gov/files/press /exhibits/dream-speech.pdf.

15. History.com. (2009). March on Washington. *A+E Networks*. Available from http://www.history.com/topics/black-history/march-on-washington.

16. Goodreads. Martin Luther King, Jr., Quotes. Available from http://www.goodreads.com/quotes/16364-life-s-most-persistent-and-urgent-question-is -what-are-you.

17. Goodreads. Martin Luther King, Jr., Quotes. Available from http://www.goodreads.com/quotes/943-darkness-cannot-drive-out-darkness-only-light -can-do-that.

18. Haney, W. (1964). "A Comparative Study of Unilateral and Bilateral Communication." *Academy of Management Journal* 7 (2): 128–136. Available from http://www.jstor.org/stable/255021.

CHAPTER 5. THE NEED FOR CONTINUAL LEARNING

1. Undelivered remarks for Democratic State Committee. Municipal Auditorium, Austin, Texas, November 22, 1963. John F. Kennedy Presidential Library and Museum. Available from https://www.jfklibrary.org/Asset-Viewer /Archives/JFKPOF-048-023.aspx.

2. Centers for Disease Control and Prevention. About CDC 24-7. Available from https://www.cdc.gov/about/.

3. Johnson, C. W. (2000). *The Spirit of a Place Called Meharry: The Strength of Its Past to Shape the Future*. Franklin, TN: Hillsboro Press.

4. US Department of Health and Human Services. National Institutes of Health. Turning Discovery into Health. Bethesda, MD. Available from https:// www.nih.gov/.

5. US Department of Education. Federal Student Aid. StudentLoans.gov. Available from https://studentloans.gov/myDirectLoan/index.action.

6. Centers for Disease Control and Prevention. Vaccines for Children Program. Department of Health and Human Services. Available from https:// www.cdc.gov/vaccines/programs/vfc/index.html.

7. Szilagyi, P. G., S. Schaffer, L. Shone, R. Barth, S. G. Humiston, M. Sandler, and L. E. Rodewald. (2002). "Reducing Geographic, Racial, and Ethnic Dispari- ties in Childhood Immunization Rates by Using Reminder/Recall Interventions in Urban Primary Care Practices." *Pediatrics* 110 (5): e58. Available from http:// pediatrics.aappublications.org/content/110/5/e58.short.

8. Lockheed Martin. Our History. Available from http://www.lockheedmartin .com/us/100years/timeline.html.

9. Schmidt, E. "In memoriam: Dr. Sherman Mellinkoff Led UCLA School of Medicine as Dean for Record 24 Years," July 21, 2016. UCLA Newsroom. Available from http://newsroom.ucla.edu/releases/in-memoriam:-dr-sherman -mellinkoff-led-ucla-school-of-medicine-as-dean-for-record-24-years.

10. Care International. Available from http://www.care-international.org/.

CHAPTER 6. A THREE-DIMENSIONAL PERSPECTIVE ON LEADERSHIP

1. "Meharry Medical College Is Troubled by Deepening Financial Crisis." *New York Times News Summary*. March 4, 1981. A12, 4–6. Available from http:// www.nytimes.com/1981/03/04/nyregion/news-summary-wednesday-march-4 -1981.html.

2. US Department of Health and Human Services. *Healthy People 2010: Understanding and Improving Health*, 2nd ed. Washington, DC: US GPO Office, November 2000. Available from https://www.healthypeople.gov/2010/document /pdf/uih/2010uih.pdf.

3. Green, M. S. (2004). "Abraham Lincoln and Civil War America: A Biography, by William E. Gienapp; Abraham Lincoln, by Thomas Keneally; Abraham Lincoln and a Nation Worth Fighting For, by James A. Rawley." *Journal of the Abraham Lincoln Association* 25 (2): 90–98. Available from http://quod.lib.umich.edu/j/jala/2629860.0025.209?view=text;rgn=main.

4. Shmoop editorial team. (November 11, 2008). "Franklin D. Roosevelt in World War II." Shmoop. Shmoop University, Inc. Available from http://www.shmoop.com/wwii/franklin-d-roosevelt.html.

5. Office of the Historian. "U.S.-Soviet Relations, 1981–1991." Available from https://history.state.gov/milestones/1981–1988/u.s.-soviet-relations.

6. History.com. "Barack Obama." Available from http://www.history.com/topics/us-presidents/barack-obama.

7. Holan, A. G. August 18, 2009. "Number of Those without Health Insurance about 46 Million." Available from http://www.politifact.com/truth-o-meter/statements/2009/aug/18/barack-obama/number-those-without-health-insurance-about-46-mil/.

8. Fluker, W. E. (2009). *Ethical Leadership: The Quest for Character, Civility, and Community.* Minneapolis, MN: Fortress Press.

9. History.com. (2009; updated 2019). Civil Rights Movement. *A+E Network.* Available from http:www.history.com/topics/black-history/civil-rights-movement.

CHAPTER 7. DISCIPLINE IN THE QUEST FOR HEALTH EQUITY

1. Bruhn, J. G. (2014). "Understanding Health Disparities." In *Culture and Health Disparities*. SpringerBriefs in Public Health. Springer, Cham. Available from https://link.springer.com/chapter/10.1007/978-3-319-06462-8.

2. Watts, Los Angeles. (n.d.). In Wikipedia. Available from https://en.wikipedia.org/wiki/Watts,_Los_Angeles.

3. 100 Black Men of America, Inc. Our History. Available from: http://www.100blackmen.org/history/.

4. Institute of Medicine Committee for the Study of the Future of Public Health. (1988). *The Future of Public Health.* Washington, DC: National Academies Press. doi: 10.17226/1091. Available from https://www.ncbi.nlm.nih.gov/books/NBK218214/?report=reader.

5. US Department of Health and Human Services. *Physical Activity and Health: A Report of the Surgeon General.* Atlanta, GA: HHS, Centers for Disease Control and Prevention, National Center for Chronic Disease Prevention and Health Promotion, 1996.

6. Satcher, D. Keynote Address to the American Pharmaceutical Association. Washington, D.C., March 13, 2000.

7. US Department of Health, Education, and Welfare. *Smoking and Health: Report of the Advisory Committee to the Surgeon General of the Public Health Service.* Washington, DC: US Department of Health, Education, and Welfare, Public Health Service, Center for Disease Control, 1964. PHS Publication No. 1103.

8. US Department of Health and Human Services. *The Health Consequences of Smoking—50 Years of Progress. A Report of the Surgeon General.* Atlanta, GA: HHS, Centers for Disease Control and Prevention, National Center for Chronic Disease Prevention and Health Promotion, Office on Smoking and Health, 2014.

9. Mayo Clinic Staff. (2016). "Stress Symptoms: Effects on Your Body and Behavior." Available from http://www.mayoclinic.org/healthy-lifestyle/stress -management/in-depth/stress-symptoms/art-20050987.

Chapter 8. Leading from Science to Policy to Practice

1. US Department of Agriculture and Nutrition Service. National School Lunch Program. Background and Development. Available from https://www.fns .usda.gov/nslp/history#1.

2. US Department of Agriculture and Nutrition Service. Team Nutrition: Local School Wellness Policy. Available from http://www.fns.usda.gov/tn/local -school-wellness-policy.

3. S. 2507, 108th Congress. Child Nutrition and WIC Reauthorization Act of 2004. Available from https://www.govtrack.us/congress/bills/108/s2507.

4. US Department of Agriculture and Nutrition Service. School Meals: Healthy Hunger-Free Kids Act of 2010. Available from http://www.fns.usda.gov /school-meals/healthy-hunger-free-kids-act.

5. Story, M., M. S. Nanney, and M. B. Schwartz. (2009). "Schools and Obesity Prevention: Creating School Environments and Policies to Promote Healthy Eating and Physical Activity." *Milbank Quarterly* 87 (1): 71–100. http:// doi.org/10.1111/j.1468-0009.2009.00548.x Available from https://www.ncbi.nlm .nih.gov/pmc/articles/PMC2879179/.

6. Lee, S. M., C. R. Burgeson, J. E. Fulton, and C. G. Spain. (2006). "Physical Education and Physical Activity: Results from the School Health Policies and Programs Study, 2006." *J Sch Health* 77 (8): 435–463. [PubMed]. Available from https://www.ncbi.nlm.nih.gov/pubmed/17908102/.

7. US Department of Health and Human Services. Reports of the Surgeon General, US Public Health Service. Available from https://www.surgeongeneral .gov./library/reports/index.html.

8. US Department of Health, Education, and Welfare. *Smoking and Health:*

Report of the Advisory Committee to the Surgeon General of the Public Health Service. Washington, DC: US Department of Health, Education, and Welfare, Public Health Service, Center for Disease Control, 1964. PHS Publication No. 1103.

9. Warner, K. E., and L. M. Goldenhar. (1989). "The Cigarette Advertising Broadcast Ban and Magazine Coverage of Smoking and Health." *J Public Health Policy* 10 (1): 32–42. Available from https://www.ncbi.nlm.nih.gov/pubmed /2715337.

10. American Lung Association. Smokefree Air Laws. (March 8, 2019). Available from https://www.lung.org/our-initiatives/tobacco/smokefree-environ ments/smokefree-air-laws.html.

11. American Nonsmokers' Rights Foundation. States, Commonwealths, and Municipalities with 100% Smoke Free Laws in Non-Hospitality Workplaces, Restaurants, or Bars as of January 2, 2017. Available from http://www.no-smoke .org/goingsmokefree.php?id=519.

12. Yasgur, B. S. (2014). "'Not for My Child': Dealing with Vaccine-Refusing Parents." *Medscape.* September 19. Available from http://www.medscape.com /viewarticle/830705.

13. Oakley, G. P., Jr. (2009). "The Scientific Basis for Eliminating Folic Acid-Preventable Spina Bifida: A Modern Miracle from Epidemiology." *Ann Epidemiol* 19: 226–230. Available from: https://www.ncbi.nlm.nih.gov/pubmed /19344858

14. Centers for Disease Control and Prevention, Folic Acid Research. Division of Birth Defects. National Center on Birth Defects and Developmental Disabilities. Available from https://www.cdc.gov/ncbddd/folicacid/research.html.

15. Crider, K. S., L. B. Bailey, and R. J. Berry. (2011). "Folic Acid Food Fortification—Its History, Effect, Concerns, and Future Directions." *Nutrients* 3 (3): 370–384. Available from https://www.ncbi.nlm.nih.gov/pmc/articles /PMC3257747/.

16. Commission on Social Determinants of Health. *Closing the Gap in a Generation: Health Equity through Action on the Social Determinants of Health.* Final report of the CSDH. Geneva: World Health Organization, 2008.

17. Moore, L., and A. Roux. (2006). "Associations of Neighborhood Characteristics with the Location and Type of Food Stores." *American Journal of Public Health* 96: 325–331.

18. Treuhaft, S., and A. Karpyn. (2010). "The Grocery Gap: Who Has Access to Healthy Food and Why It Matters." *PolicyLink.* Available from http://thefood trust.org/uploads/media_items/grocerygap.original.pdf.

19. Flournoy, R. (2006). "Healthy Foods, Strong Communities: Fresh Fruits and Veggies Are Good for More Than Just Your Health." National Housing

Institute. Issue #143. Available from http://www.nhi.org/online/issues/147 /healthyfoods.html.

20. H.R. 3590: Patient Protection and Affordable Care Act. 111th Congress, 2009–2010 Public Law No: 111–148. March 23, 2010. Available from https:// www.congress.gov/bill/111th-congress/house-bill/3590.

21. Learn about the Affordable Care Act. Available from http://hhs.gov /healthcare/about-the-aca/index.html.

22. US Department of Health and Human Services. *Healthy People 2020: Topics and Objectives*. Washington, DC, October: 2019. Available from https:// www.healthypeople.gov/2020/topics-objectives.

23. McKinlay, J. B. (1995). *The New Public Health Approach to Improving Physical Activity and Autonomy in Older Populations, in Preparation for Aging*, ed. E. Heikkinen. New York: Plenum Press, 87–103.

24. Health Project. Johnson & Johnson Services, Inc. (2019). Available from http://thehealthproject.com/winner/johnson-johnson-services-inc-johnson -johnson-health-and-wellness/.

25. Satcher, D. Keynote Address to the American Pharmaceutical Association. Washington, D.C., March 13, 2000.

26. US Department of Health and Human Services. *Women and Smoking: A Report of the Surgeon General*. Rockville (MD): HHS, Public Health Service, Office of the Surgeon General, 2001.

27. Cockburn, D., and D. Deapen, eds. (2004). *Cancer Incidence and Mortality in California: Trends by Race/Ethnicity, 1988–2001*. Los Angeles Cancer Surveillance Program, University of Southern California. Available from http://www .ccrcal.org/pdf/Reports/CCRMonograph12-04_2.pdf.

28. National Institutes of Health, National Institute on Minority Health and Health Disparities. "Satcher Health Leadership Institute Creates New Generation of Parent Leaders." Available from https://www.nimhd.nih.gov/news-events /features/2014/satcher-health-leadership.html.

29. CDC Foundation: Helping CDC Do More, Faster. What Is Public Health? Available from http://www.cdcfoundation.org/content/what-public -health.

30. Institute of Medicine. (1988). *The Future of Public Health*. Washington, DC: National Academies Press. doi:10.17226/1091. Available from https://www .nap.edu/read/1091/chapter/1.

31. 90 by 30. The Public Health Approach to Prevention. (2013). University of Oregon College of Education. Available from https://90by30.com/our -philosophy/public-health-approach-prevention.

32. Satcher, D., G. E. Fryer, J. McCann, A. Troutman, S. H. Woolf, and

G. Rust. (2005). "What If We Were Equal? A Comparison of the Black-White Mortality Gap in 1960 and 2000." *Health Affairs* 24: 459–464.

33. McGinnis, J. M., and W. H. Foege. (1993). "Actual Causes of Death in the United States." *JAMA* 270 (18): 2207–2212. doi:10.1001/jama.1993 .03510180077038. Available from http://jamanetwork.com/journals/jama/article -abstract/409171.

34. US Department of Health and Human Services. *Healthy People 2010.* Washington, DC: HHS, January; 2000. Available from www.health.gov/healthy people/.

35. CDC/National Center for Health Statistics. *Healthy People 2020.* Available from https://www.cdc.gov/nchs/healthy_people/hp2020.htm.

36. Ford Foundation. (2002). Annual Report, 2002, p. 52. Available from https://fordfoundcontent.blob.core.windows.net/media/1529/ar2002.pdf.

37. US Department of Health and Human Services. Office of the Surgeon General; Office of Population Affairs. *The Surgeon General's Call to Action to Promote Sexual Health and Responsible Sexual Behavior.* Rockville, MD: OSG, July 2001.

38. Focus on the Family. Helping Families Thrive. Available from http:// www.focusonthefamily.com/.

39. SIECUS. About Us. Available from https://siecus.org/about-siecus/.

40. American Academy of Pediatrics. Dedicated to the Health of All Children. Available from https://www.aap.org/en-us/about-the-aap/aap-facts/Pages /AAP-Facts.aspx.

41. The National Consensus Process on Sexual Health and Responsible Sexual Behavior. Interim Report, 2006. Available from http://www.msm.edu /Files/CESH_NCP_Interim Report.pdf.

42. Hatcher, R., S. Rachel, and C. Thrasher. (2016). *Sexual Etiquette 101 & More.* Atlanta, GA: Managing Contraception, LLC.

43. Van Vogt, M. "5 Big Ideas about the Origins of Homosexuality: The Genetics of Gayness." *Psychology Today,* December 29, 2012. Available from https://www.psychologytoday.com/blog/naturally-selected/201212/5-big-ideas -about-the-origins-homosexuality.

44. World Health Organization. Emergencies Preparedness, Response. Smallpox. Available from http://www.who.int/csr/disease/smallpox/en/.

45. Weir, H. K., R. N. Anderson, S. M. Coleman King, A. Soman, T. D. Thompson, Y. Hong, B. Moller, et al. (2016). "Heart Disease and Cancer Deaths— Trends and Projections in the United States, 1969–2020." *Prev Chronic Dis* 13: 160211. Available from https://www.cdc.gov/pcd/issues/2016/16_0211.htm.

46. American Diabetes Association. (2006). "Trends in Death Rates among U.S. Adults with and without Diabetes between 1997 and 2006: Findings from the National Health Interview Survey." *Diabetes Care* 39 (12). Available from http://care.diabetesjournals.org/content/35/6/1252.

47. US Department of Health and Human Services. *The Health Consequences of Smoking: A Report of the Surgeon General*. Atlanta, GA: HHS, Centers for Disease Control and Prevention, National Center for Chronic Disease Prevention and Health Promotion, Office on Smoking and Health, 2004.

48. US Department of Health and Human Services. *Preventing Tobacco Use among Youth and Young Adults: A Report of the Surgeon General*. Atlanta, GA: HHS, Centers for Disease Control and Prevention, National Center for Chronic Disease Prevention and Health Promotion, Office on Smoking and Health, 2012.

49. H.R. 1256: Family Smoking Prevention and Tobacco Control Act. 111th Congress, 2009. Available from https://www.govtrack.us/congress/bills/111/hr1256.

50. US Department of Health and Human Services. *The Health Consequences of Smoking—50 Years of Progress: A Report of the Surgeon General*. Atlanta, GA: HHS, Centers for Disease Control and Prevention, National Center for Chronic Disease Prevention and Health Promotion, Office on Smoking and Health, 2014.

51. History.com. (2009). Nixon Signs Legislation Banning Cigarette Ads on Television and Radio. *A+E Network*. Available from http://www.history.com/this-day-in-history/nixon-signs-legislation-banning-cigarette-ads-on-tv-and-radio.

52. CDC Newsroom. "Cigarette Smoking among US Adults Lowest Ever Recorded: 14% in 2017." Available from http://cdc.gov/media/releases/2018/p1108-cigarette-smoking-adults.html.

53. World Health Organization. History of the World Health Organization Framework Convention on Tobacco Control. 2009. Available from http://apps.who.int/iris/handle/10665/44244.

54. World Health Organization. Tobacco Free Initiative. *WHO Global Report on Trends in Tobacco Smoking, 2000–2025*. Available from http://www.who.int/tobacco/publications/surveillance/reportontrendstobaccosmoking/en/.

55. US Department of Health and Human Services. *Physical Activity and Health: A Report of the Surgeon General*. Atlanta, GA: HHS, Centers for Disease Control and Prevention, National Center for Chronic Disease Prevention and Health Promotion, 1996; US Department of Health and Human Services. *The Surgeon General's Call to Action to Prevent and Decrease Overweight and Obesity*. Rockville, MD: HHS, Public Health Service, Office of the Surgeon General, July 2001.

CHAPTER 9. CONFRONTING THE EPIDEMIC OF OVERWEIGHT
AND OBESITY

1. Hruby, A., and F. B. Hu. (2015). "The Epidemiology of Obesity: A Big Picture." *PharmacoEconomics* 33 (7): 673–689. http://doi.org/10.1007/s40273 -014-0243-x. Available from: https://www.ncbi.nlm.nih.gov/pmc/articles /PMC4859313/.

2. Centers for Disease Control and Prevention. *Principles of Epidemiology in Public Health Practice: An Introduction to Applied Epidemiology and Biostatistics*, 3rd ed. (updated May 26, 2012). Available from https://www.cdc.gov/ophss/csels /dsepd/ss1978/lesson1/section11.html.

3. US Department of Health and Human Services. *The Surgeon General's Call to Action to Prevent and Decrease Overweight and Obesity.* Rockville, MD: HHS, Public Health Service, Office of the Surgeon General, 2001.

4. Brennan, V. M., ed. *Journal of Health Care for the Poor and Underserved.* Johns Hopkins University Press. Available from http://www.press.jhu.edu /journals/journal_of_health_care_for_the_poor_and_underserved/guidelines .html.

5. Action for Healthy Kids, Annual Report, 2005–2006. Available from http://www.actionforhealthykids.org/storage/documents/AFHK_Annual _Report_2005-2006_FINAL.pdf.

6. US Department of Health and Human Services. *Physical Activity and Health: A Report of the Surgeon General.* Atlanta, GA: HHS, Centers for Disease Control and Prevention, National Center for Chronic Disease Prevention and Health Promotion, 1996.

7. US Department of Agriculture and Nutrition Service. Team Nutrition. Local School Wellness Policy. Available from http://www.fns.usda.gov/tn/local -school-wellness-policy.

8. US Department of Agriculture and Nutrition Service. National School Lunch Program. Available from http://www.fns.usda.gov/nslp/whats-new.

9. GENYOUth. GenYouth: Exercise Your Influence. Available from http:// www.genyouthnow.org/about-us.

10. Fuel Up to Play 60. Available from https://www.fueluptoplay60.com /about/about-the-program.

11. Georgia SHAPE. Available from http://www.georgiashape.org/.

12. Community Voices at Morehouse School of Medicine. Available from https://communityvoices.org/.

13. Berry, L. L., A. M. Mirabito, and W. B. Baun. (2010). "What's the Hard Return on Employee Wellness Programs?" *Harvard Business Review.* Available

from https://hbr.org/2010/12/whats-the-hard-return-on-employee-wellness
-programs.

14. Satcher, D. Keynote Address to the American Pharmaceutical Association. Washington, D.C., March 13, 2000.

15. Breedlove, N. "Sodium: The Silent Killer of African Americans." *Huffing-
ton Post* (updated May 2015). Available from http://www.huffingtonpost.com
/nicole-breedlove/sodium-the-silent-killer-of-african-americans_b_4937023
.html#.

16. Katz, D. L., and A. Ali. *Preventive Medicine, Integrative Medicine, and the
Health of the Public*. Commissioned for the Institute of Medicine, February 2009.
Available from http://researchgate.net/publication/237429179_Preventive
_medicine_integrated_medicine_and_the_health_of_the_public.

17. Commission on Social Determinants of Health. *Closing the Gap in a
Generation: Health Equity through Action on the Social Determinants of Health*.
Final report of the CSDH. Geneva: World Health Organization, 2008.

CHAPTER 10. THE ADVANCEMENT OF REPRODUCTIVE HEALTH

1. Institute of Medicine. (1988). *The Future of Public Health*. Washington, DC:
National Academies Press. doi:10.17226/1091.

2. Health 24. "The Menstrual Cycle from Menarche to Menopause."
February 24, 2011. Available from http://www.health24.com/Lifestyle/Woman
/Menstruation/The-menstrual-cycle-from-menarche-to-menopause-20120721.

3. Nove, A., Z. Matthews, S. Neal, and A. V. Camacho. (2014). "Maternal
Mortality in Adolescents Compared with Women of Other Ages: Evidence from
144 Countries." *Lancet Global Health* 2 (3): 155–164. Available from https://www
.thelancet.com/journals/langlo/article/PIIS2214-109X(13)70179-7/abstract?
code=lancet-site.

4. World Health Organization. *News release*. "United Nations Agencies
Report Steady Progress in Saving Mothers' Lives." May 6, 2014. Available from
http://www.who.int/mediacentre/news/releases/2014/maternal-mortality/en/.

5. MacDorman, M. F., T. J. Mathews, A. D. Mohangoo, and J. Zeitlin. (2014).
"International Comparisons of Infant Mortality and Related Factors: United
States and Europe, 2010." *National Vital Statistics Reports* 63 (5). Hyattsville, MD:
National Center for Health Statistics, 2014.

6. List of Countries by Infant Mortality Rates. (2016). In Wikipedia. Available from https://en.wikipedia.org/wiki/List_of_countries_by_infant_mortality
_rate#UN_Bermuda.

7. Roser, M. (2017). "Child Mortality." Published online at OurWorldInData

.org. Available from https://ourworldindata.org/child-mortality/ [Online Resource]. Data source: UN Inter-agency Group for Child Mortality Estimation (IGME). Link: http://childmortality.org.

8. Commission on Social Determinants of Health. *Closing the Gap in a Generation: Health Equity through Action on the Social Determinants of Health.* Final report of the CSDH. Geneva: World Health Organization, 2008.

9. DataBlog. "Maternal Mortality: How Many Women Die in Childbirth in Your Country?" *Guardian.* 2010. Available from https://www.theguardian.com /news/datablog/2010/apr/12/maternal-mortality-rates-millennium-development -goals#data.

10. Points of Light. About Points of Light. Available from http://www.points oflight.org/about-us/.

11. UNICEF for Every Child. Available from https://www.unicef.org/.

12. Henry Kaiser Family Foundation. (2000). LoveLife. The Foundation's Largest Initiative Ever Aims to Curb HIV Infection among South African Youth. Available from http://www.kff.org/other/lovelife/.

13. CNN.com. "U.S., South Africa Plan to Improve Trade, Fight Crime." February 18, 1999. Available from http://www.cnn.com/WORLD/africa/9902/18 /us.sa.talks/.

14. Malan, M. "SA Has Highest Number of New HIV Infections Worldwide— Survey," April 1, 2014. Available from http://bhekisisa.org/article/2014-04-01-sa -holds-highest-number-of-new-hiv-infections-worldwide-survey.

15. Jehl, D. "Surgeon General Forced to Resign by White House." *New York Times.* December 10, 1994. Available from http://www.nytimes.com/1994/12/10 /us/surgeon-general-forced-to-resign-by-white-house.html.

16. US Department of Health and Human Services. Office of the Surgeon General, Office of Population Affairs. *The Surgeon General's Call to Action to Promote Sexual Health and Responsible Sexual Behavior.* Rockville, MD: OSG, July 2001. Available from http://www.ncbi.nlm.nih.gov/books/NBK44216/.

17. Stobbe, M. (2014). *Surgeon General's Warning: How Politics Crippled the Nation's Doctor.* Oakland: University of California Press.

18. HIV.gov. PEPFAR: PEPFAR and Global AIDS. Available from https:// www.hiv.gov/federal-response/pepfar-global-aids/pepfar.

19. The National Consensus Process on Sexual Health and Responsible Sexual Behavior. Interim report. 2006. Available from http://www.msm.edu /Files/CESH_NCP_Interim Report.pdf.

20. Hatcher, R., S. Rachel, and C. Thrasher. *Sexual Etiquette 101 & More.* Atlanta, GA: Managing Contraception, LLC, 2016.

21. US Department of Health and Human Services. *Tobacco Use among U.S.*

Racial/Ethnic Minority Groups—African Americans, American Indians and Alaska Natives, Asian Americans and Pacific Islanders, and Hispanics: A Report of the Surgeon General. Atlanta, GA: HHS, Centers for Disease Control and Prevention, National Center for Chronic Disease Prevention and Health Promotion, Office on Smoking and Health, 1998.

22. US Department of Health and Human Services. *Reducing Tobacco Use: A Report of the Surgeon General*. Atlanta, GA: HHS, Centers for Disease Control and Prevention, National Center for Chronic Disease Prevention and Health Promotion, Office on Smoking and Health, 2000.

23. US Department of Health and Human Services, Public Health Service, Office of the Surgeon General, *Women and Smoking: A Report of the Surgeon General*. Atlanta, GA: US Centers for Disease Control and Prevention, Office of Smoking and Health, 2001.

24. US Department of Health and Human Services. *Oral Health in America: A Report of the Surgeon General*. Rockville, MD: HHS, National Institute of Dental and Craniofacial Research, National Institutes of Health, 2000.

25. US Department of Health and Human Services. *The Surgeon General's Call to Action to Prevent and Decrease Overweight and Obesity*. Rockville, MD: HHS, Public Health Service, Office of the Surgeon General, 2001.

26. *The Health Consequences of Smoking—50 Years of Progress. A Report of the Surgeon General*. Atlanta, GA: US Department of Health and Human Services, Centers for Disease Control and Prevention, National Center for Chronic Disease Prevention and Health Promotion, Office on Smoking and Health, 2014.

27. US Department of Health, Education, and Welfare. *Smoking and Health: Report of the Advisory Committee to the Surgeon General of the Public Health Service*. Washington, DC: US Department of Health, Education, and Welfare, Public Health Service, Center for Disease Control, 1964. PHS Publication No. 1103.

28. US Department of Health and Human Services. *Mental Health: A Report of the Surgeon General*. Rockville, MD: HHS, Substance Abuse and Mental Health Services Administration, Center for Mental Health Services, National Institutes of Health, National Institute of Mental Health, 1999.

29. US Public Health Service, *Report of the Surgeon General's Conference on Children's Mental Health: A National Action Agenda*. Washington, DC: HHS, 2000. Stock No. 017-024-01659-4 ISBN No. 0-16-050637-9.

30. US Department of Health and Human Services. *Mental Health: Culture, Race, and Ethnicity—A Supplement to Mental Health: A Report of the Surgeon General*. Rockville, MD: HHS, Substance Abuse and Mental Health Services Administration, Center for Mental Health Services, 2001.

31. Shands, K. N., G. P. Schmid, B. B. Dan, D. Blum, R. J. Guidotti, N. T. Hargrett, R. L. Anderson, et al. (1980). "Toxic Shock Syndrome in Menstruating Women: Association with Tampon Use and Staphylococcus aureus and Clinical Features in 52 Cases." *N Engl J Med* 303: 1436–1442.

32. Centers for Disease Control and Prevention. National Center for HIV/ AIDS, Viral Hepatitis, STD, and TB Prevention. Available from https://www.cdc .gov/nchhstp/default.htm.

33. The Gates Foundation. Available from https://www.gatesfoundation.org/.

34. CARE. Unprecedented Times Call for Unprecedented Generosity. Available from https://my.care.org/site/Donation2?df_id=21546&21546.

35. McKinsey & Company. "A New CEO for McKinsey Social Initiative." Available from: http://www.mckinsey.com/about-us/new-at-mckinsey-blog /a-new-ceo-for-the-mckinsey-social-initiative.

36. Oakley, G. P., Jr. (2009). "The Scientific Basis for Eliminating Folic Acid–Preventable Spina Bifida: A Modern Miracle From Epidemiology." *Ann Epidemiol* 9: 226–230. Available from https://www.ncbi.nlm.nih.gov/pubmed /19344858.

37. Centers for Disease Control and Prevention. (2016). Office of the Director. "Seven Decades of Firsts with Seven CDC Directors." Available from https://www.cdc.gov/cdcgrandrounds/pdf/2016_july_phgr_poster_gerberding _web.pdf.

38. Commission on Social Determinants of Health. *Closing the Gap in a Generation: Health Equity through Action on the Social Determinants of Health.* Final report of the CSDH. Geneva: World Health Organization, 2008.

Chapter 11. Overcoming the Stigma of Mental Health Problems

1. US Department of Health and Human Services. *Mental Health: A Report of the Surgeon General—Executive Summary.* Rockville, MD: HHS, Substance Abuse and Mental Health Services Administration, Center for Mental Health Services, National Institutes of Health, National Institute of Mental Health, 1999.

2. Borus, J. F., M. J. Howes, N. P. Devins, R. Rosenberg, and W. W. Livingston. (1988). "Primary Health Care Providers' Recognition and Diagnosis of Mental Disorders in Their Patients." *Gen Hosp Psychiatry* 10: 317–321. Available from https://www.ncbi.nlm.nih.gov/pubmed/3169532.

3. Kennedy, P., and S. Fried. *A Common Struggle: A Personal Journey through the Past and Future of Mental Illness and Addiction.* New York: Blue Rider Press, 2016.

4. National Alliance of Mental Illness (NAMI). Jailing People with Mental Illness. 2017. Available from https://www.nami.org/Learn-More/Public-Policy /Jailing-People-with-Mental-Illness.

5. The Mental Health Parity and Addiction Equity Act of 2008. The Center for Consumer Information and Insurance Oversight. Available at https://www .cms.gov/CCIIO/Programs-and-Initiatives/Other-Insurance-Protections/mhpaea _factsheet.html.

6. CNN.com/Inside Politics. Sunday, December 29, 2002. "Senator, Family Members Killed in Minnesota Plane Crash." Available from http://www.cnn .com/2002/ALLPOLITICS/10/25/plane.crash.minn/.

7. Community Mental Health Act. (February 16, 2017). In Wikipedia. Available from https://en.wikipedia.org/w/index.php?title=Community_Mental _Health_Act&oldid=765722808.

8. Kennedy, P. J. "Kennedy: Mental Health Is Civil Rights Issue of Today." *Las Cruces Sun News*. September 17, 2016. Available from https://www.lcsun-news .com/story/opinion/commentary/2016/09/17/kennedy-mental-health-civil-rights -issue-today/90576458/.

9. Householder, M. "Actress Glenn Close Aims to Reduce Mental Health Stigma." March 29, 2018. Available from https://kitv.com/story/37843820 /actress-glenn-close-aims-to-reduce-mental-health-stigma.

10. Ushistory.org. (2016). The Sit-In Movement. *US History Online Textbook*. Available from http://www.ushi.story.org/us/54d.asp.

11. Learn about the Affordable Care Act. Available from http://hhs.gov /healthcare/about-the-aca/index.html.

12. History.com. (2009; updated 2019). Civil Rights Movement. *A+E Network*. Available from http:www.history.com/topics/black-history/civil-rights -movement.

13. The Kennedy Forum: State of the Union in Mental Health and Addiction. Available from https://www.thekennedyforum.org/events/stateoftheunion.

14. McKee, A. C., R. C. Cantu, C. J. Nowinski, E. Tessa-Hedley-Whyte, B. E. Gavett, A. E. Budson, V. E. Santini, et al. (2009). "Chronic Traumatic Encephalopathy in Athletes: Progressive Tauopathy following Repetitive Head Injury." *Journal of Neuropathology and Experimental Neurology* 68 (7): 709–735. Available from: https://www.ncbi.nlm.nih.gov/pmc/articles/PMC2945234/.

15. National Council on Youth Sports Safety. Available from https://www .idealist.org/en/nonprofit/fdafb2a4317040949a9360546b629993-national -council-on-youth-sports-safety-inc-atlanta.

16. Centers for Disease Control and Prevention. National Center for Injury Prevention and Control. Traumatic Brain Injury and Concussion. TBI: Get the

Facts. 2017. Available from https://www.cdc.gov/traumaticbraininjury/get_the
_facts.html.

17. National Federation of State High School Associations. "Recommendations and Guidelines for Minimizing Head Impact Exposure and Concussion
Risk in Football." Report from the July 2014 NFHS Concussion Summit Task
Force. Available from https://www.nfhs.org/media/1014885/2014_nfhs
_recommendations_and_guidelines_for_minimizing_head_impact_october
_2014.pdf.

18. Gaba, A. (2014). "The Culture of Mental Health Stigma in Communities
of Color." Robert Wood Johnson Foundation: Culture of Health. Available from
http://www.rwjf.org/en/culture-of-health/2014/05/the_culture_of_mental.html.

19. Chow, JC-C., K. Jaffee, and L. Snowden. (2003). "Racial/Ethnic Disparities in the Use of Mental Health Services in Poverty Areas." *American Journal of
Public Health* 93 (5): 792–797. Available from https://www.ncbi.nlm.nih.gov
/pmc/articles/PMC1447841/.

20. Suicide Prevention Resource Center. (2013). *Suicide among Racial/Ethnic
Populations in the U.S.: American Indians/Alaska Natives*. Waltham, MA: Education
Development Center. Available from https://www.samhsa.gov/capt/sites/default
/files/resources/suicide-ethnic-populations.pdf.

21. Okafor, M., G. Wrenn, V. Ede, N. Wilson, W. Custer, E. Risby, M. Claeys,
et al. (2016). "Improving Quality of Emergency Care through Integration of
Mental Health." *Community Mental Health Journal* 52: 332–342. Available from
https://www.ncbi.nlm.nih.gov/pubmed/26711094.

22. National Institute of Mental Health. "Transforming the Understanding
and Treatment of Mental Illnesses: Integrated Care." Available from https://
www.nimh.nih.gov/health/topics/integrated-care/index.shtml.

23. Hwang, W., J. Chang, M. LaClair, and H. Paz. (2013). "Effects of Integrated Delivery System on Cost and Quality." *Am J Manag Care* 19 (5): e175–e184.
Available from http://www.ajmc.com/journals/issue/2013/2013-1-vol19-n5/effects
-of-integrated-delivery-system-on-cost-and-quality.

24. Rust, G., K. Kondwani, R. Martinez, R. Dansie, W. Wong, Y. Fry-Johnson,
and H. Strothers. (2006). "A CRASH-Course in Cultural Competence." *Ethnicity
& Disease* 16: 29–36. [*PubMed*].

25. Office of the Surgeon General; Center for Mental Health Services;
National Institute of Mental Health. *Mental Health: Culture, Race, and Ethnicity:
A Supplement to Mental Health: A Report of the Surgeon General*. Rockville, MD:
Substance Abuse and Mental Health Services Administration, August 2001.
Available from https://www.ncbi.nlm.nih.gov/books/NBK44243/.

26. Nelson, A. R., A. Y. Stith, and B. D. Smedley, eds. (2002). *Unequal

Treatment: Confronting Racial and Ethnic Disparities in Health Care [full printed version]. Washington, DC: National Academies Press.

27. Harris, R., and E. Ofili. The Satcher Health Leadership Institute's Transdisciplinary Collaborative Center for Health Disparities. Available from http://msm.edu/Research/research_centersandinstitutes/SHLI/TCC/index.php.

28. Insel, T. (May 15, 2015). Post by Former NIMH Director Thomas Insel: Mental Health Awareness Month: By the Numbers. Available from https://www.nimh.nih.gov/about/directors/thomas-insel/blog/2015/mental-health-awareness-month-by-the-numbers.shtml.

29. Jamison, K. R. (1996). *An Unquiet Mind*. New York: Vintage Books.

30. National Institute of Mental Health. "Children and Mental Health." Available from https://www.nimh.nih.gov/health/publications/treatment-of-children-with-mental-illness-fact-sheet/index.shtml.

31. Tynan, W. D., K. Woods, and J. Carpenter. American Psychological Association. "Integrating Child Psychology Services in Primary Care." Available from http://www.apa.org/pi/families/resources/primary-care/integrating-services.aspx.

CHAPTER 12. LEADERSHIP BEYOND EXPERTISE

1. Forsyth. (June 13, 2017). Former Surgeon General Dr. David Satcher Awarded the Forsyth Icon in Health Award at Discover Forsyth: A Taste & a Toast to Good Health. Available from https://forsyth.org/news/former-surgeon-general-dr-david-satcher-awarded-forsyth-icon-health-award-discover-forsyth#.Xa9zvJJKjIU.

2. US Department of Health and Human Services. *Oral Health in America: A Report of the Surgeon General*. Rockville, MD: HHS, National Institute of Dental and Craniofacial Research, National Institutes of Health, 2000.

3. HHS.gov. "About the Epidemic: The U.S. Opioid Epidemic." (June 15, 2017). Available from https://www.hhs.gov/opioids/about-the-epidemic/index.html#m.

4. History.com. (2009). "Columbine High School Shootings." *A+E Networks*. Available from http://www.history.com/topics/columbine-high-school-shootings.

5. SAMHSA. About Us. Available from https://www.samhsa.gov/about-us.

6. CDC. About CDC 24–7. [Last updated, July 13, 2017]. Available from https://www.cdc.gov/about/default.htm.

7. Office of the Surgeon General; National Center for Injury Prevention and Control; National Institute of Mental Health; Center for Mental Health Services. *Youth Violence: A Report of the Surgeon General*. Rockville, MD: OSG, 2001. Available from https://www.ncbi.nlm.nih.gov/books/NBK44294/.

8. Centers for Disease Control and Prevention. Injury Prevention and Control: Funded Injury Control Research Centers (ICRCs). Available from https://www.cdc.gov/injury/erpo/icrc/index.html.

9. NPR. "Jay Dickey, Arkansas Congressman Who Blocked Gun Research, Dies at 77." April 24, 2017. Available from http://www.npr.org/2017/04/25/525604434/jay-dickey-arkansas-congressman-who-blocked-gun-research-dies-at-77.

10. Dickey, J., and M. Rosenberg. (July 27, 2012). "We Won't Know the Cause of Gun Violence until We Look for It" [opinion]. Available from https://www.washingtonpost.com/opinions/we-wont-know-the-cause-of-gun-violence-until-we-look-for-it/2012/07/27/gJQAPfenEX_story.htm.

11. Durbin, D. "Durbin Calls for End to Ban on Centers for Disease Control Gun Violence Research." [Press Release], January 14, 2016. Available from https://www.durbin.senate.gov/newsroom/press-releases/durbin-calls-for-end-to-ban-on-centers-for-disease-control-gun-violence-research.

12. US Department of Health and Human Services. *The Surgeon General's Call to Action to Prevent and Decrease Overweight and Obesity*. Rockville, MD: HHS, Public Health Service, Office of the Surgeon General, July, 2001. Available from US GPO, Washington, DC.

13. *The Face of a Child: Surgeon General's Workshop and Conference on Children and Oral Health*. (May 2001). Available from https://www.nidcr.nih.gov/Data Statistics/SurgeonGeneral/Conference/ConferenceChildrenOralHealth/Documents/SGR_Conf_Proc.pdf.

14. US Department of Health, Education, and Welfare. *Smoking and Health: Report of the Advisory Committee to the Surgeon General of the Public Health Service*. Washington, DC: US Department of Health, Education, and Welfare, Public Health Service, Center for Disease Control, 1964. PHS Publication No. 1103.

15. US Department of Health and Human Services. History of the Office of the Surgeon General. Available from http://www.surgeongeneral.gov/about/history/index.html.

16. US Public Health Service. Office of the Surgeon General. Office of the Assistant Secretary for Health. *Healthy People: The Surgeon General's Report on Health Promotion and Disease Prevention*. Washington, DC: US Department of Health, Education, and Welfare, Public Health Service, 1979. Publication No. 79-55071.

17. US Department of Health and Human Services. *Healthy People 2010: Understanding and Improving Health*, 2nd ed. Washington, DC: US GPO, November 2000.

18. US Department of Health and Human Services. Commissioned Corps of

the US Public Health Service. America's Health Responders. Available from https://coausphs.org/page/Americas_Health_responsders.

19. National Research Council and Institute of Medicine Panel on Needle Exchange and Bleach Distribution Programs. (1994). *Proceedings Workshop on Needle Exchange and Bleach Distribution Programs*. Washington, DC: National Academies Press. "Assessing the Efficacy of Needle Exchange Programs: An Epidemiological Perspective." Available from https://www.ncbi.nlm.nih.gov/books/NBK236637/.

20. US Department of Health and Human Services. NIH Almanac. Harold D. Varmus, MD. Available from https://www.nih.gov/about-nih/what-we-do/nih-almanac/harold-e-varmus-md.

21. National Institute of Allergy and Infectious Disease. Anthony S. Fauci, MD, NIAID Director. Available from https://www.niaid.nih.gov/about/director.

22. National Library of Medicine. "Meet Local Legend: Vivian Pinn, M.D." Available from https://wayback.archive-it.org/org-350/20190508153142/https://www.nlm.nih.gov/exhibition/locallegends/Biographies/Pinn_Vivian.html.

CHAPTER 13. THE TEAM APPROACH TO LEADERSHIP

1. "Meharry Medical College Is Troubled by Deepening Financial Crisis." *New York Times News Summary*. March 4, 1981, A12, 4–6. Available from http://www.nytimes.com/1981/03/04/nyregion/news-summary-wednesday-march-4-1981.html.

2. Johnson, C. W. (2000).*The Spirit of a Place Called Meharry: The Strength of Its Past to Shape the Future*. Franklin, TN: Hillsboro Press.

3. Esty, K., R. Griffin, and M. S. Hirsch. (1995). *Workplace Diversity*. Avon, MA: Adams Media Corporation.

4. Taylor, B. "Why Sports Are a Terrible Metaphor for Business." *Harvard Business Review*. February 2017. Available from https://hbr.org/2017/02/why-sports-are-a-terrible-metaphor-for-business.

5. Maxwell, J. (2013). *How Successful People Lead*. New York: Center Street.

6. Covey, S. (1989). *The Seven Habits of Highly Successful People*. New York: Free Press.

7. Collins, J. C. (2001). *Good to Great: Why Some Companies Make the Leap and Others Don't*. New York: Harper Business.

8. Fluker, W. E. (2009). *Ethical Leadership: The Quest for Character, Civility, and Community*. Minneapolis, MN: Fortress Press.

CHAPTER 14. LEADING FOR INSTITUTIONAL SUSTAINABILITY

1. "Run with Purpose, Finish with Pride." Available from http://www.marinemarathon.com/.

2. National Medical Association. About Us. (n.d.). Available from http://www.nmanet.org/page/About_Us.

3. American Medical Association. History. (n.d.). Available from https://www.ama-assn.org/ama-history.

4. *JAMA* (journal). (September 13, 2017). In Wikipedia. Available from https://en.wikipedia.org/wiki/JAMA (journal).

5. Lawson, W. (n.d.). Journal of the National Medical Association. Available from: https://www.sciencedirect.com/journal/journal-of-the-national-medical-association

6. Centers for Medicare & Medicaid Services. "History." (2019). Available from https://www.cms.gov/About-CMS/Agency-Information/History/index.html.

7. Thurgood Marshall College Fund. "Historically Black Colleges and Universities." (n.d.). Available from https://tmcf.org/about-us/our-schools/brief-history-of-hbcus.

8. History.com. (2010; updated 2019). This Day in History. "University of Alabama Desegregated." Available from: http://www.history.com/this-day-in-history/university-of-alabama-desegregated.

9. History.com. (2009; updated 2019). Civil Rights Movement. *A+E Network*. Available from http:www.history.com/topics/black-history/civil-rights-movement.

10. HBCU Money. Our Money Matters. Available from https://hbcumoney.com/2017/02/06/2016-top-10-hbcu-endowments/.

11. C. W. Johnson. (2000). *The Spirit of a Place Called Meharry: The Strength of Its Past to Shape the Future*. Franklin, TN: Hillsboro Press.

12. NPR. (March 1, 2017). Code Switch. Race and Identity, Remixed. "HBCUs Graduate More Poor Black Students than White Colleges." Available from http://www.npr.org/sections/codeswitch/2017/03/01/517770255/hbcus-graduate-more-poor-black-students-than-white-colleges.

13. UNICEF for Every Child. Available from https://www.unicef.org/what-we-do.

14. US AID. (n.d.). PEPFAR Strategy for Accelerating HIV/AIDS Epidemic Control. (2017–2020). Available from https://aidsfree.usaid.gov/news-events/news/pepfar-strategy-accelerating-hivaids-epidemic-control-2017-2020.

15. Rotary: People of Action. (n.d.). Available from https://www.rotary.org/.

Index

Academy of Family Medicine, 121
access, to health care, 40, 43–44, 105; for
  mental illness, 45, 140–43, 147–48, 153
Action for Healthy Kids, 115–16
adolescents: pregnancy, 126, 128–29, 132,
  136–37, 189; sexual health education,
  129–32; sports-related concussions, 144–45
Affordable Care Act (ACA), 14, 45–46, 102,
  142–43
Africa: HIV/AIDS epidemic, 129–30, 131–32,
  137, 189–90; reproductive health care,
  128–30, 137, 189
African American(s): hypertension risk, 122;
  mental illness treatment, 145; mortality
  rates, 38
African American medical school students, 48,
  186–87
African American men, adverse social
  conditions, 39
African American women: disrespect towards,
  26–28; mortality rates, 39
aging, healthy, 97
American Academy of Pediatrics, 106
American Association of Medical Colleges,
  186–87
American Medical Association (AMA),
  180–82
American Nurses Association, 34
American Psychological Association, 152–53
American Society of Pediatrics, 121
Anniston, AL, 4–5, 20, 21, 82, 183, 187

Arthur Blank Foundation, 118
Asian Americans, 145
Atlanta, GA, civil rights movement in, 7, 8, 10,
  22–23, 24, 25, 71, 142
Atlanta Braves, 118
Atlanta Falcons, 118
Atlanta University Center, 2, 6–7, 24, 70–71,
  73, 74

Banda, Hastings K., 128, 189
Bare, John, 118
behavior, as social determinant of health, 40,
  43–44, 97, 105, 120, 124
Betts, Virginia, 34
Blair, Tony, 34
board of trustees, leader's relationship with,
  51–52, 53–55
Boner, Bill, 52–53
Boston University, 86
brain injuries, sports-related, 143–45, 175
Broome, Claire, 31–32, 134–35
Bush, George H. W., 42, 129
Bush, George W., 41–42, 131–32, 136

Calhoun County Training School, Hobson City,
  AL, 21, 183
California, anti-smoking regulations, 100, 103,
  108
cancer, 11, 37, 107, 122
cardiovascular disease, 38, 107, 108, 109, 114,
  122, 133